Endometrial Adenocarcinoma: Prevention and Early Diagnosis

Monographs in Clinical Cytology

Vol. 17

Series Editor

Svante R. Orell Kent Town

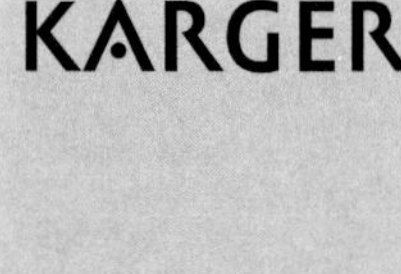

Endometrial Adenocarcinoma

Prevention and Early Diagnosis

Matías Jiménez-Ayala Madrid
Beatriz Jiménez-Ayala Portillo Madrid

Including contributions by

Enrique Iglesias Goy Madrid
Mar Rios Vallejo Madrid

176 figures, 171 in color, and 40 tables, 2008

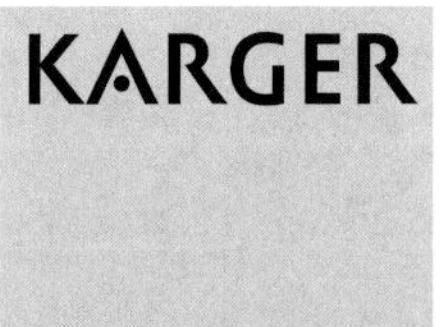

Basel · Freiburg · Paris · London · New York ·
Bangalore · Bangkok · Singapore · Tokyo · Sydney

· ·

Endometrial Adenocarcinoma: Prevention and Early Diagnosis

Dr. Matías Jiménez-Ayala, MD, FIAC, Past-President of the IAC
Dr. Beatriz Jiménez-Ayala Portillo, MD, MIAC
Instituto Jiménez-Ayala
C/ Hermosilla, 126
E-28028 Madrid (Spain)
E-Mail matiasjimenezayala@hotmail.com

Enrique Iglesias Goy, MD, Director of Department of Obstetric and Gynecology,
Universidad Autónoma, Madrid, Spain
Mar Rios Vallejo, MD, Department of Obstetric and Gynecology, Hospital
Universitario Puerta de Hierro, Madrid, Spain

Library of Congress Cataloging-in-Publication Data

Jiménez-Ayala, Matías.
    Endometrial adenocarcinoma : prevention and early diagnosis / Matías
Jiménez-Ayala, Beatriz Jiménez-Ayala Portillo ; including contributions by
Enrique Iglesias Goy, Mar Rios Vallejo.
        p. ; cm. – (Monographs in clinical cytology, ISSN 0077-0809 ; vol.
17)
    Includes bibliographical references and index.
    ISBN 978-3-8055-8480-7 (hard cover : alk. paper)
    1. Endometrium–Cancer.   2. Endometrium–Cancer–Cytodiagnosis.   3.
Adenocarcinoma–Cytodiagnosis.   I. Jiménez-Ayala Portillo, Beatriz.   II.
Title.   III. Series.
    [DNLM: 1. Carcinoma, Endometrioid.   2. Endometrium–cytology.   W1 MO567KF
v.17 2008 / WP 460 J61e 2008]
    RC280.U8.J56 2008
    616.99′465–dc22
                                                        2008001900

To Maria José, our wife and mother, for her support and help in our cytopathological work
Matías Jiménez-Ayala and Beatriz Jiménez-Ayala Portillo

Contents

Contents

Chapter 10

Cytopathology of the Non-Epithelial Malignant Tumors of the Uterine Corpus

Preface

Endometrial adenocarcinoma is the most common malignant tumor of the female genital tract in developed countries and its incidence has increased over recent years.

Over the past 35 years the authors have gained considerable experience in endometrial cytology and with the different techniques for obtaining this material, including being the first to use the Medhosa cannula. The Spanish Society of Cytology recommended a nomenclature for reporting endometrial cytology following the Bethesda System in 1990.

At the 15th International Congress of Cytology, Santiago de Chile, 2004, Dr. Matías Jiménez-Ayala chaired a Panel devoted to: 'Endometrial Adenocarcinoma: Prevention and Early Diagnosis' with the participation of Dr. A. Castiglioni (Chile), Dr. E. Iglesias (Spain), Dr. J. Whitaker and B. Knight (South Africa) and Dr. T. Jobo (Japan). Dr. Svante Orell encouraged us to write a monograph on this subject in Karger's series *Monographs in Clinical Cytology*. A previous monograph on endometrial cytology written by J.W. Reagan and A.B.P. Ng (1989) has been out of print for many years. The current policy in the prevention and early diagnosis of endometrial cancer is to direct screening programs to selected risk populations using cytologic, histopathologic and some gynecologic techniques such as transvaginal sonography and hysteroscopy. These techniques and the various presentations of benign and malignant diseases of the endometrium are presented by a team of authors: Dr. Enrique Iglesias, an acknowledged expert in the above gynecological techniques, a young cytopathologist, Dr. Beatriz Jiménez-Ayala, and a senior expert on endometrial cytology, Dr. Matías Jiménez-Ayala.

We hope that our monograph proves to be useful to cytopathologists, pathologists interested in diseases of the female genital tract, cytotechnologists and students of the above professional areas of pathology.

Acknowledgement

We would like to thank Dr. Svante Orell, the inspirator behind this monograph, for his support and help throughout the preparation of this book.

We gratefully acknowledge the cooperation of staff of the Instituto Jiménez-Ayala, especially Concha Chinchilla, our senior CTIAC, and Paloma Fernández Rueda for her hard and efficient secretarial work. We also thank Manuel Nevado and Miguel López de la Riva for their contributions of several figures of ESS and endometrial polyp.

Dr. Matías Jiménez-Ayala, FIAC Past-President of the IAC.
Dr. Beatriz Jiménez-Ayala Portillo, MIAC.

Foreword

The incidence of endometrial cancer is increasing – particularly in industrialized countries – thought to be due to a combination of factors including hormonal imbalance (hyperestrinism), obesity and aging of the population. In contrast to the cervix, where cytologic screening has been enormously successful in preventing cervical cancer, there is no effective general population screening of asymptomatic women for endometrial cancer. Most endometrial adenocarcinomas present with symptoms of postmenopausal bleeding triggering evaluation of the uterine cavity.

A variety of collection techniques are available to obtain cytologic or histopathologic samples for diagnosis. However, interpretation of such specimens can be difficult without proper collection and preparation. Thankfully, this monograph provides a most valuable educational resource for the pathologist and cytopathologist in the techniques of endometrial sampling and diagnosis.

Dr. Matias Jiménez-Ayala, senior author of the monograph, is an internationally recognized cytopathologist with over 90 publications in the field. In 1993, he received the Maurice Goldblatt award for his lifetime contributions to cytology. He is past president of the International Academy of Cytology, Past President and Honorary President of the Spanish Society of Cytology and an honorary member of the Argentine, Brazilian, Chilean, Mexican, and Uruguayan Societies of Cytology, Latin America, as well as the Portuguese Society of Cytology. For this monograph, Dr. Jiménez-Ayala has drawn on his 35 years of experience in endometrial sampling and endometrial cytopathology. He is ably accompanied in this effort by his daughter Beatriz Jiménez-Ayala, an accomplished cytopathologist in her own right. Drs. Enrique Iglesias and Maria Rios Vallejo have contributed an informative chapter on vaginal ultrasound and hysteroscopy for endometrial assessment.

The chapters are comprehensive and logically organized, covering the epidemiology and pathogenesis of endometrial adenocarcinoma, endometrial sampling techniques and the spectrum of cytomorphologic appearance from benign through hyperplasia to adenocarcinoma of the endometrium. A separate chapter covers non-epithelial uterine malignancies. Throughout the monograph, inclusion of both cytologic and H&E histologic images allows cytohistologic correlation of lesions.

In summary, this is a welcome addition to Karger's series of *Monographs in Clinical Cytology*. This contribution will bring clarity to a difficult area of cytodiagnosis and will become an important reference text on the shelves of cytopathology laboratories.

Diane Solomon, MD
President-Elect, International Academy of Cytology
Bethesda, Md.

···

List of Abbreviations

AEC	Atypical endometrial cells		EnA	Endometrioid adenocarcinoma
AEH	Atypical endometrial hyperplasia		EnC	Endocervical cells
AGC	Atypical glandular cells		EP	Endometrial polyp
AGUS	Atypical glandular cells of undetermined significance		ESC	Eosinophilic syncytial change
			ESS	Endometrial stromal sarcoma
AH	Atypical hyperplasia		ETh	Endometrial thickness
AIS	Adenocarcinoma in situ of endocervix		HPV	Human papillomavirus
ASC	Atypical squamous cells		HRT	Hormone replacement therapy
ASCCP	American Society of Colposcopy and Cervical Pathology		HSIL	High-grade squamous intraepithelial lesions
			IUD	Intrauterine device
ASC-H	Atypical squamous cells, cannot exclude high-grade squamous intraepithelial lesion		IUMC	Indiana University Medical Center
			LBP	Liquid-based preparation
ASC-US	Atypical squamous cells of undetermined significance		LMS	Leiomyosarcoma
			LUS	Lower uterine segment
CBP	Cell block preparation		MA	Mucinous adenocarcinoma
CCA	Clear-cell adenocarcinoma		MMMT	Malignant mixed mesodermal tumor
CLEA	Clear-cell endometrial adenocarcinoma		MMT	Malignant mesenchymal tumor
CIN	Cervical intraepithelial neoplasia		MRI	Magnetic resonance imaging
CIS	Carcinoma in situ		OC	Oral contraceptive
COC	Combined oral contraceptives		Pap	Pap smear
CP	Conventional preparation		PI	Index of pulse
CT	Computed tomography		PSCCE	Primary squamous cell carcinoma of the endometrium
CVS	Cervicovaginal smear			
D&C	Dilatation of the cervix and curettage		RI	Index of resistance
DUB	Dysfunctional uterine bleeding		SmCC	Small cell carcinoma
EA	Endometrial adenocarcinoma		SEA	Serous endometrial adenocarcinoma
EBT	Endometrial brushing techniques		SERM	Selective estrogen receptor modulators
EC	Endometrial carcinoma		TAM	Tamoxifen
ECA	Endocervical adenocarcinoma		TBS	The Bethesda System
ECG	Endometrial Collaborative Group		TP	Thin-Prep
EH	Endometrial hyperplasia		TS	Transvaginal sonography
EIN	Endometrial intraepithelial neoplasia		UES	Undifferentiated endometrial sarcoma
EMs	Endometrial cells		UPSC	Papillary serous carcinoma of the uterus
EN	Endometrioid neoplasia			

 List of Abbreviations

Current Status of the Prevention and Early Diagnosis of Endometrial Adenocarcinoma

1.1. Epidemiology

Increasing Incidence of Endometrial Adenocarcinoma
Endometrial adenocarcinoma (EA) is the most common malignant tumor of the female genital tract in developed countries, where 80–85% of cases are estrogen-dependent tumors and 15–20% are non-estrogen-dependent (WHO, 2003).

The incidence of EA has increased in industrialized countries over the last 20 years (USA, Northern Europe, Japan) [64, 83, 193]. In most regions in Spain, the incidence is higher than that of carcinoma of the uterine cervix. In France, the prevalence of EA is at an intermediate level, between 13.6 and 24/100,000 [115]. Current epidemiological data from Japan [101] confirms that the incidence of endometrial carcinoma (EC) is increasing whereas that of cervical carcinoma is decreasing slightly. Forty years ago, 5% of uterine cancers were ECs, recently the proportion of EC had risen to more than 40%. Most patients are between 50 and 59 years of age but the incidence is increasing in all age groups. The Japanese group found that the increase in the incidence of EC in Japan is due to three growing risk factors: obesity, larger numbers of nulliparous and elderly women, and an increase in the average life span of Japanese women from 53.96 years in 1947 to 88.23 years in 2003. Finally, they predict that the number of patients with EC in Japan will grow from 892 in 1975 to 6,623 in 2015 [101].

Geographic Factors, Race, Age and Occupational Exposure
Geographic Factors and Fat Consumption. The incidence of EC varies considerably from one country to another. It is generally lower in third world nations and higher in more industrialized countries, suggesting a relation to fat consumption. Women 9.09–22.7 kg above their ideal body weight have a threefold increased risk of EC when compared to age-matched controls; women >22.7 kg above their ideal body weight have a ninefold increased risk of EA [85].

EA is the most common genitourinary malignancy in women in the USA. There are 33,000 new cases each year, more than twice the number of cervical cancers [222]. American women over the age of 45 tend to have a higher risk of EC than of cervical cancer [64].

The incidence of EA in white women in southern USA tends to be higher than in women from the north and west [55].

Race. In the USA, incidence rates for endometrial malignant tumors are lower in blacks than in whites, but mortality rates are higher in blacks [188]. The survival rate for black women has remained constant at 30–40% for the last 30 years. The survival rate for white women was 80–85% in the same period [64]. Figures from the Cancer Registry suggest that this racial imbalance is attributable to a higher incidence of low-grade tumors in white women, possibly due to differences in exogenous hormone use, more common in white women. In addition, the rare aggressive tumors are more frequent in black women [37, 188].

Age. The median age of patients at the time of diagnosis of EA is 63 years. The incidence of EA is highly dependent on age, 12 cases per 100,000 women at 40 years of age compared to 84 cases per 100,000 at 60 years of age [56, 85]. EC is a more aggressive neoplasm in elderly patients than in the general population due to the higher proportion of cancers with non-endometrioid histology, which are usually diagnosed at a later stage. Holfman et al. [80] found only 57% endometrioid type tumors in the older age group compared to 75–80% in the general population. Nulliparity and infertility are significantly more frequent in young patients with EA.

Poor prevention and late detection of aggressive tumors in elderly patients necessitate great efforts to encourage women to seek medical attention early when symptoms first appear.

Occupational Exposure. EC has been associated with exposure to animal dust and sedentary work [220].

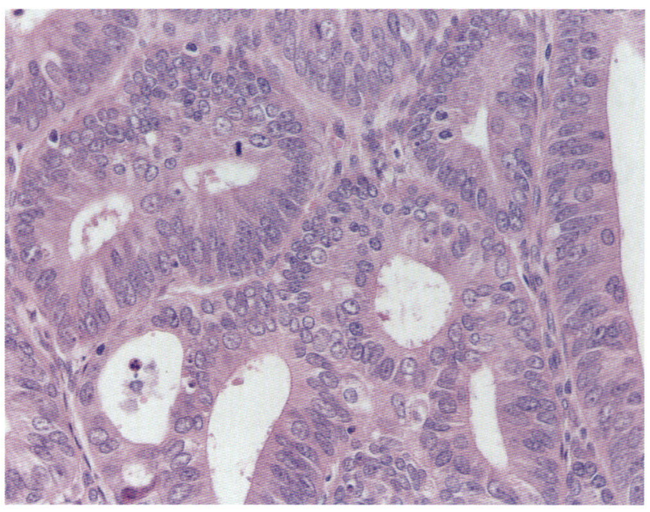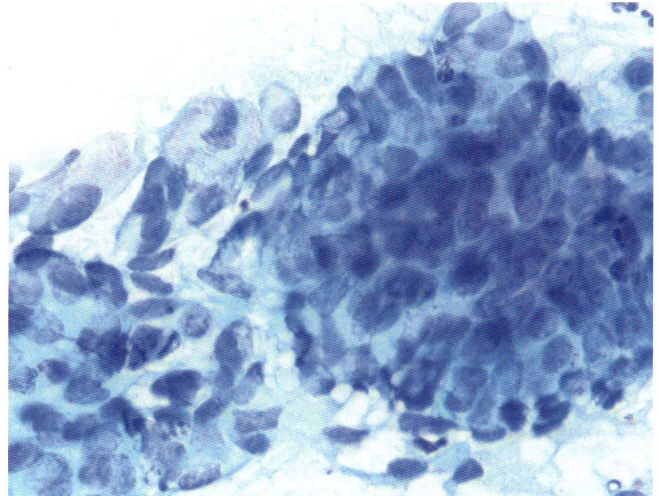

Fig. 1.1. Endometrial adenocarcinoma type I, low grade. **a** Histopathology: HE, 20×; **b** cytology: Pap, 60×.

Viral Agents Human Papillomavirus

Infection with specific human papillomavirus (HPV) types has been implicated in the development of cervical, vaginal and vulvar cancers. Several authors have postulated that EC, mostly with squamous components, may have an HPV-related etiology [184]. The apparent association of low-risk HPV types (types 6 and 11) with benign squamous elements and high-risk types (types 16, 18, 31 and 33) with malignant elements [20, 161] is intriguing, but requires further studies. Some authors [46] think that the endometrium may not be a suitable host epithelium for HPV replication and maturation.

1.2. Pathogenesis

EC is a biologically and histologically diverse group of neoplasms with differing pathogenesis. Estrogen-dependent carcinomas (type I) are low grade (fig. 1.1) and frequently associated with endometrial hyperplasia (EH), in particular atypical hyperplasia. Unopposed estrogenic stimulation is the driving force behind anovulatory cycles, occurring in women with polycystic ovaries or at the time of menopause. The iatrogenic use of unopposed estrogen as hormone replacement therapy (HRT) is a predisposing factor for EC. The second type of EC (type II) appears to be less related to sustained estrogenic stimulation [193] (fig. 1.2).

1.3. Hormonal Therapy. The Effects on the Endometrium

Hormonal Replacement Therapy and Contraceptives. It has been accepted that the use of exogenous estrogens influences the development of EC. The effect appears to be less if estrogens are associated with progestagen [133]. The incidence of EC in the USA peaked around 1975 after a significant increase in the late 1960s consequent to the extended use of unopposed estrogens in HRT. As soon as progestogens were added and the use of unopposed estrogens was decreased, a significant decrease in the incidence of EC was noted [64]. A Northern European study [17] found that the long cycle HRT modality with a progestin administered over 10 days every 12 weeks may increase the risk of EH and eventually of cancer, compared to conventional HRT with a monthly cycle. Careful monitoring of the endometrium is recommended, especially if the long cycle HRT modality is used.

Combined Oral Contraceptives (COC). During the past 45 years, COC have become a key component of modern fertility regulation programs. In recent years, 100 million women throughout the world are estimated to be using this method of contraception [75].

Virtually all the studies investigating COC and EC have found a lower risk among current or past users [75]. The overall reduction in EC risk is about 40–50% with stronger effects among long-term users. The protection persists for up to 20 years after COC are discontinued. This protective effect is also related to the age at first use and the period of time since last use [88]. This mainly benefits women at risk of developing estrogen-dependent carcinoma (type I), the most common of these tumors, but the incidence also seems lower for type II, the more aggressive EC [85]. Figures from a registry for EC in young women taking oral contraceptives (OC) showed that the majority of these patients received sequential OC [62].

Current Status of the Prevention and Early
Diagnosis of Endometrial Adenocarcinoma

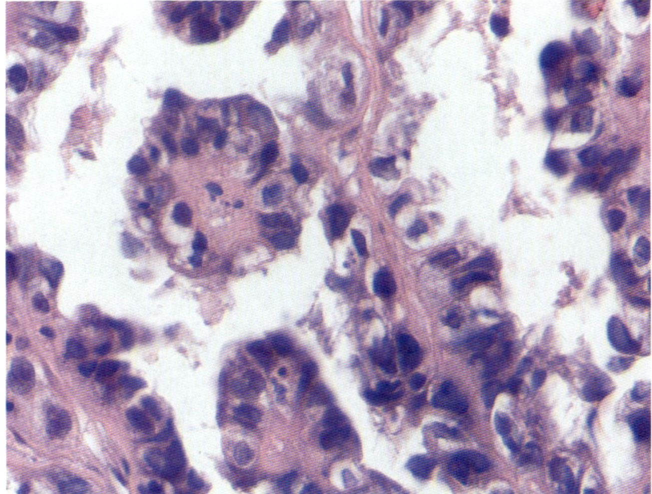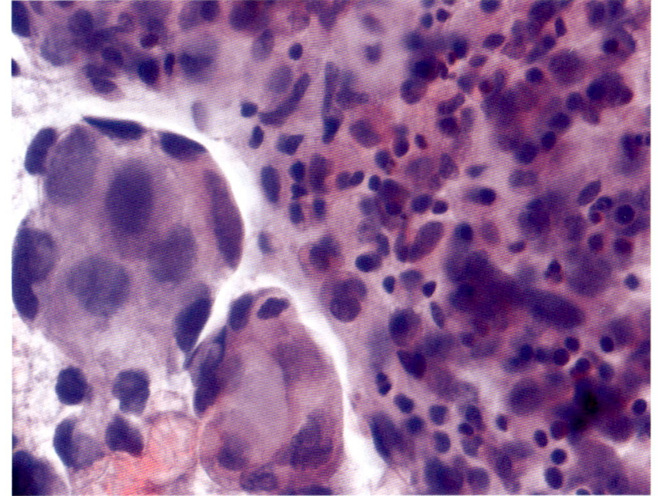

Fig. 1.2. Endometrial adenocarcinoma type II, serous papillary adenocarcinoma. **a** Histopathology: HE, 40×; **b** cytology: Pap, 60×.

Most published evidence relates to older high estrogen dose OC. There is less information on the effects of currently available low-dose 'pills' on EC.

Finally, there seems to be no evidence of an association between synthetic diethylstilbestrol DES and the risk of endometrial and ovarian cancer, although there is a known association with clear cell adenocarcinoma of the vagina [207].

Endometrial Pathology and Breast Cancer

Coadjuvant Therapy with Tamoxifen

Tamoxifen (TAM) is a selective estrogen receptor modulator (SERM)[1], it is believed to perform its antitumor action as an anti-estrogenic, but the drug also has mixed estrogenic and anti-estrogenic effects on the estrogen receptors that varies between target organs [7].

Endometrial pathology has been identified in up to 36% of postmenopausal breast cancer TAM-treated patients [36].

As TAM causes an increased incidence of both premalignant and malignant lesions of the endometrium [26], the International Agency for Research on Cancer has classified TAM as an endometrial carcinogen.

Other SERMs with potentially greater antitumor efficacy and an attenuated uterotrophic profile are being investigated, but TAM remains the principal therapy for treatment and prevention of breast cancer. Newer hormonal therapies, including other SERMs[1], pure anti-estrogens and aromatase inhibitors, are likely to have more selective applications [10].

[1]Selective estrogen receptors modulators.

To decrease the risk of EC, the duration of TAM therapy should be limited to the shortest period of accepted efficacy.

Endometrial Polyp and Hyperplasia

Endometrial polyp (EP) represents the most common endometrial pathology associated with menopausal TAM exposure, with a high risk of malignant change (fig. 1.3–1.5, 1.9). There is no correlation between malignant change in EP and EP size and duration of treatment [36].

Proliferative endometrium is present twice as commonly in TAM-treated women than in controls. EH is 10 times more common in women treated with TAM. This finding is in agreement with ultrasonographic studies. TAM may enhance endometrial proliferation in 30–40% of postmenopausal women, but it is unclear which patients will respond to TAM as a weak estrogen and which will not [7] (fig. 1.5).

Risk of Adenocarcinoma

EH and EP, EC and malignant mixed müllerian tumors and sarcomas are more commonly diagnosed in postmenopausal TAM-treated breast cancer patients than in non-treated patients. The prognosis of EC (fig. 1.6) is worse in long-term TAM users. This seems to be due to an increased proportion of less favorable histology (clear-cell and serous carcinoma), and to higher stage. Past users had a worse prognosis with more invasive histologic features than recent users, probably due to a higher average age [74].

However, the benefits of TAM on breast cancer survival far outweigh the increased mortality from EC. Nevertheless, widespread use of TAM as a preventive agent against breast cancer in healthy women is being seriously questioned [13].

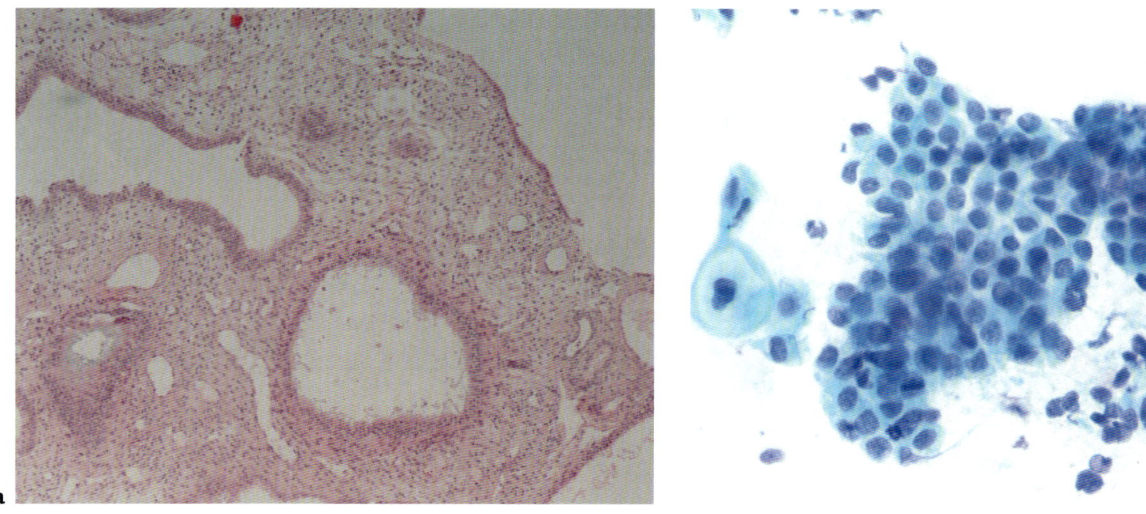

Fig. 1.3. Endometrial polyp. **a** Histopathology: HE, 4×; **b** cytology: Pap, 40×.

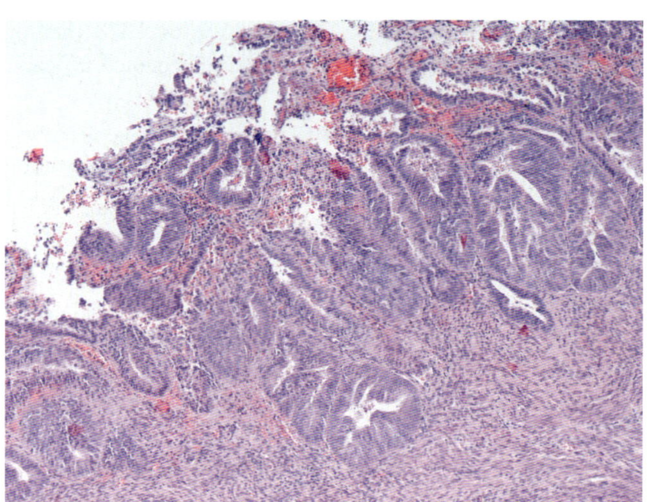

Fig. 1.4. Endometrial adenocarcinoma associated with endometrial polyp. Histopathology: HE, 10×.

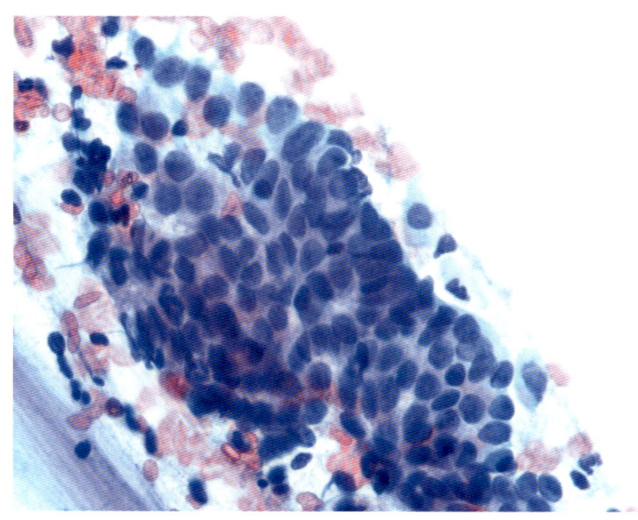

Fig. 1.5. Endometrial hyperplasia under tamoxifen. Pap, 60×.

Risk of Carcinosarcoma

The reported data supports an association between TAM therapy and the development of uterine carcinosarcoma (fig. 1.7). The risk is likely to be highest in those patients who have taken TAM for a prolonged period. The disease is in an advanced stage in most of the patients and the outcome is usually fatal [35, 119, 126].

Papillary Serous Carcinoma of the Uterus and Breast Carcinoma

Patients with papillary serous carcinoma of the uterus (UPSC) have an increased risk of development of breast cancer as compared to patients with endometrioid adenocarcinoma of the uterus. The relationship between breast and EC has not, to our knowledge, been clarified, but a close follow-up of EC patients with yearly breast examinations and mammograms is recommended, especially for those with UPSC [67] (fig. 1.8).

Management of Patients

The management of breast cancer TAM-treated patients is not yet codified: endometrial cytology, ultrasonography, hysteroscopy or endometrial biopsy are used for follow-up according to the criteria of the prescribing physician [85]. Cohen [36] and Assikis and Jordan [7] suggest annual sonography and endometrial sampling for all postmenopausal women who are being treated with TAM.

Current Status of the Prevention and Early
Diagnosis of Endometrial Adenocarcinoma

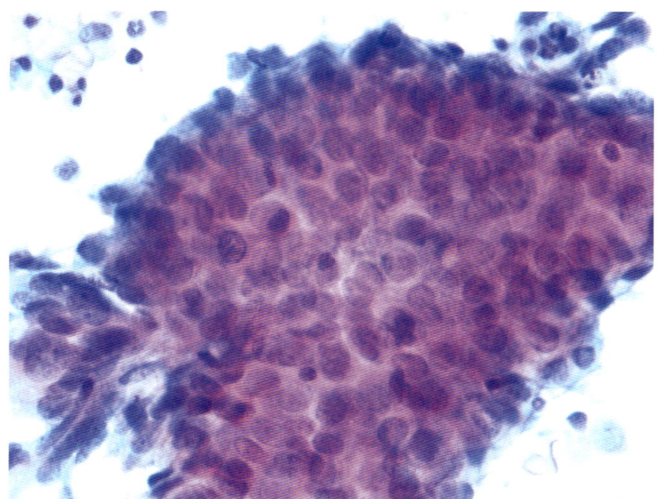

Fig. 1.6. Endometrial adenocarcinoma. Pap, 60×.

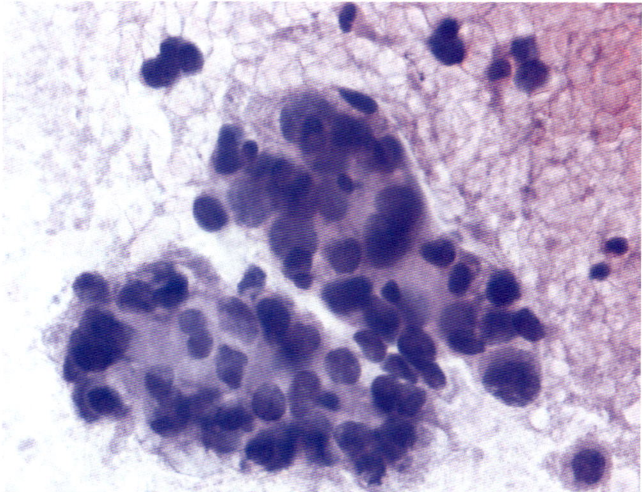

Fig. 1.8. Papillary serous carcinoma of the uterus. Pap, 60×.

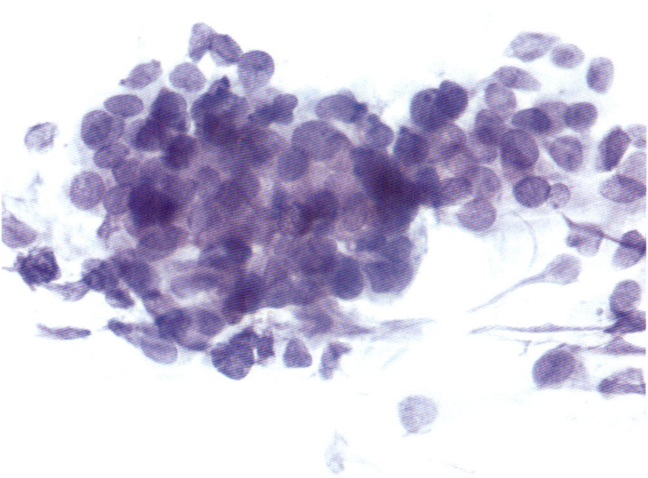

Fig. 1.7. Carcinosarcoma. Pap, 40×.

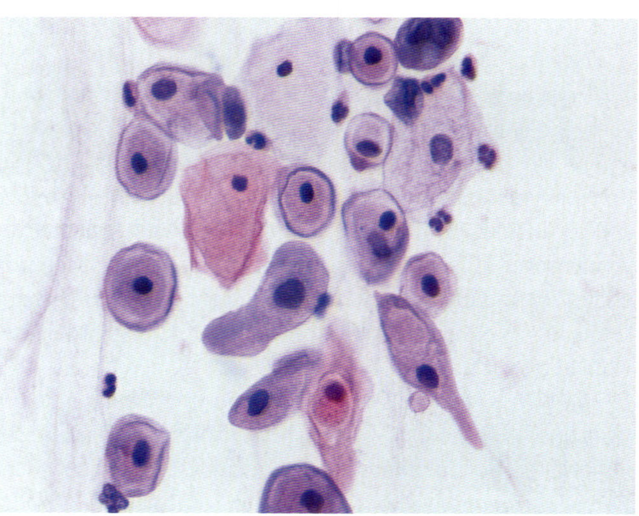

Fig. 1.9. Metaplastic reactive cells in a patient with coadjuvant therapy with tamoxifen. Pap, 40×.

Value of the Pap Smear

An individualized gynecologic evaluation based on hormonal cytology can be useful in selecting patients who will be more susceptible to TAM-induced endometrial abnormalities [189]. Particular attention should be given to the detection of endometrial cells in vaginal-cervical smears in patients who receive TAM, because these may indicate endometrial pathology [1].

In women treated with TAM there is a higher incidence of benign reactive cells (fig. 1.9) and atypical squamous cells in vaginal/cervical smears, with no increase in the risk of squamous intraepithelial lesions or cervical cancer. Small blue cells similar to reserve cells in an atrophic smear have been described. These cells are considered to be proliferative reserve cells, stimulated by the agonistic effect of TAM [163, 185]. Careful evaluation is necessary to exclude endometrial pathology as well as metastatic breast cancer (fig. 1.10).

1.4. High-Risk Population

Assessment of High-Risk Population. Epidemiological and clinical data are fundamental in establishing mass screening programs for the early detection of EC, using integrated techniques, and in defining risk groups. Such data should be taken into consideration in creating new projects [133].

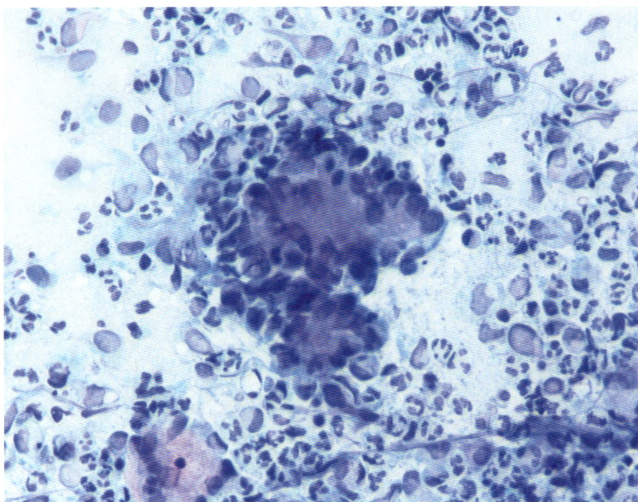

Fig. 1.10. Vaginal recurrence of endometrial adenocarcinoma with papillary area. Patient treated for breast cancer. Pap, 40×.

Prevalence of Endometrial Cancer (EC). It is important to know the prevalence of EC to decide if detection is necessary and to whom it must be directed [83]. Koss et al. [107] in 2,856 asymptomatic women found a prevalence of 0.696% and an incidence of EC of 0.171%. They suggest that all women over 50 should be screened at least once. Grönroos et al. [70] and Okamura et al. [162] agree that regular mass screening programs should be directed at asymptomatic women over 45.

High-Risk Factors. The contribution of Kurman and co-workers [193] in the WHO Classification of Tumours is important. They found that patients with estrogen-dependent EC are frequently obese, diabetic, nulliparous, hypertensive or have a late menopause. In contrast, the non-estrogen-dependent type occurs in older postmenopausal women and the tumors are high grade. Obesity is an independent risk factor, and in Western Europe it is associated with up to 40% of EC. Fat tissue predisposes obese women to uterine cancer by increasing unopposed estrogen stimulation of the endometrial lining. Tumors of the ovary, such as granulosa cell tumors, liberate estrogen and may be associated with EH and cancer [57]. Data collected from seven countries including 226 cases of EC showed no significant association between the use of an IUD and risk of EC [175].

1.5. Prevention of Uterine Cancer

Primary prevention strategies aimed at reducing the risk of ECs must initially act at the level of precursor lesions. The

Table 1.1. Diagnostic methods for endometrial screening programs

Cytology
Endometrial brushing techniques
Pathology
Office procedures: Pipelle, microbiopsy
New gynecological techniques
Transvaginal sonography
Hysteroscopy

current challenges concerning the risk of EC should be focused on: (a) risk factors including obesity, anovulation, use of unopposed estrogen therapy and TAM, nulliparity and family history of breast or colonic cancer; (b) abnormal bleeding as the most frequent sign of both cancer and its precursors, early diagnosis of these lesions is likely to improve prognosis, and (c) there is a need to develop an efficient strategy for selected screening of the high-risk population based on the above circumstances.

1.6. Population Screening Programs. Diagnostic Methods (table 1.1)

Over 90% of new cases of EC occur in women 50 years of age or older. The majority of the patients have symptoms at presentation before the diagnosis is made. There is no data to justify yearly screening for EC in low-risk populations [150]. The Spanish experience, with more than 100,000 samples obtained with various endometrial samplers, was reported during the XII International Congress of Cytology in Madrid, in May 1995, by Matías Jiménez-Ayala (the Golblatt Award Lecture [92]. Sensitivity and specificity were reported as more than 90%. The challenge is to find an adequate strategy to use in the population at high risk for EC. The current policy is to direct screening programs to selected risk populations using the following methods, which will be presented in detail in Chapters 2–5:

Cytology. We will discuss the value of the Pap smear (Pap) and of endometrial cytology.

Pathology. The endometrial sample could be taken as an office procedure: Pipelle, microbiopsies. By itself, simple endometrial biopsy cannot be used for mass screening of asymptomatic women. Endometrial cytology is far preferable, because of its easier application, even though it is less accurate for diagnosis [133].

New Gynecological Techniques. The value of transvaginal sonography and of hysteroscopy will be presented by E. Iglesias and M. Ríos.

Current Status of the Prevention and Early
Diagnosis of Endometrial Adenocarcinoma

Chapter 2

The Value of Endometrial Cytology

2.1. Types of Endometrial Cells

Exfoliated endometrial cells may be of epithelial or stromal origin, although a distinction between these two cell types is not always possible. Both types of cells, especially the epithelial endometrial cells, usually present degenerative changes that make correct identification difficult.

Epithelial endometrial cells may be present as isolated cells in a cervicovaginal smear (Pap smear), as flat sheets in brush smears. The cells are similar in size to the nuclei of intermediate squamous cells and have scant cytoplasm (fig. 2.1). More frequently, the cells occur in multi-layered aggregates, 'cell balls', and may show the pattern of the typical postmenstrual 'exodus' (fig. 2.2). Two types of stromal cells can be distinguished. Superficial stromal cells are indistinguishable from small histiocytes (fig. 2.3). Deep stromal cells are smaller, spindle or rounded, with scant cytoplasm [2, 138]. It seems that superficial stromal cells are not useful in predicting endometrial pathology [28].

2.2. The Bethesda System

Following the 2001 Bethesda Conference, The Bethesda System (TBS) terminology has been applied to the reporting of glandular abnormalities to reflect the current knowledge of glandular lesions in cervical cytology [42]. This terminology is shown in table 2.1 [138].

The 2001 glandular terminology includes some changes to the previous Bethesda reporting systems [112]:
– Atypical glandular abnormalities should be specified as to the cell of origin (endocervical or endometrial). If this is not possible, the term 'glandular' should be used.
– The term 'atypical glandular cells of undetermined significance' (AGUS) has been eliminated to avoid confusion

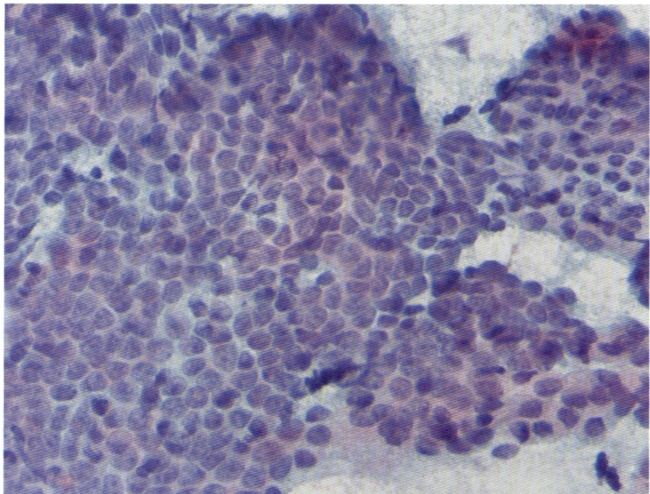

Fig. 2.1. Epithelial endometrial cells. Endometrial brushing. 40×.

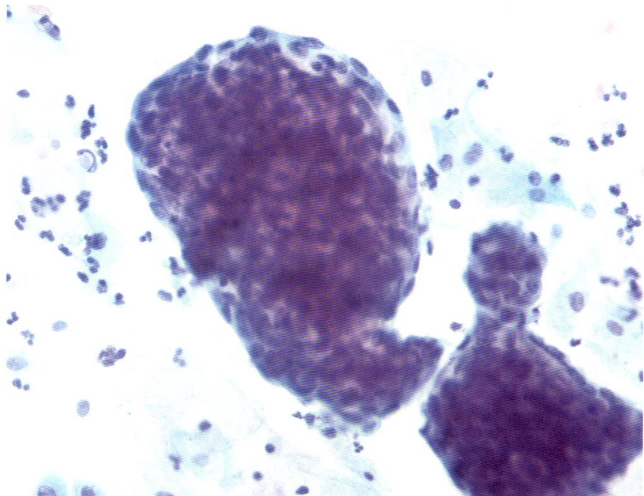

Fig. 2.2. Postmenstrual 'exodus'. Pap smear, 40×.

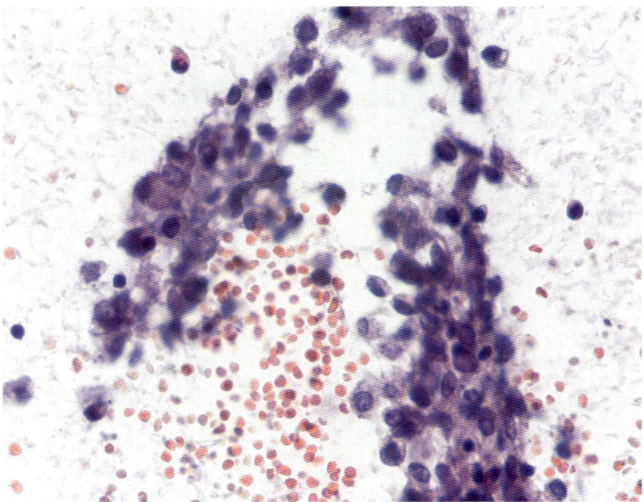

Fig. 2.3. Superficial endometrial stromal cells. Endometrial brushing. Pap, 40×.

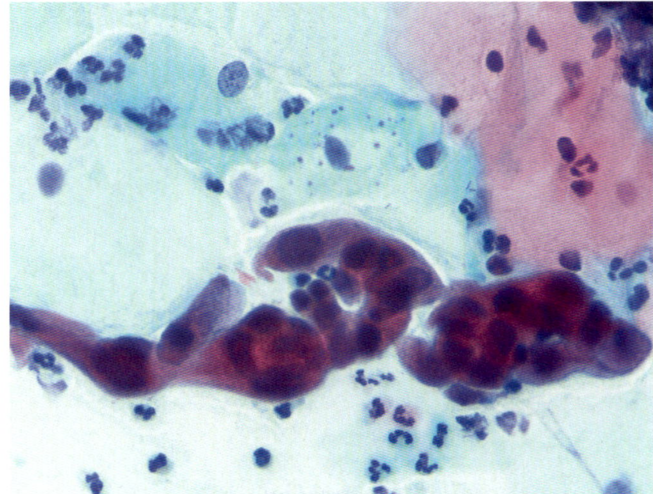

Fig. 2.4. Atypical endometrial cells. Histology: adenocarcinoma of ovary. Pap, 60×.

Table 2.1. TBS for glandular cytology

Atypical
• Endocervical cells (NOS or specify in comments)
• Endometrial cells (NOS or specify in comments)
• Glandular cells (NOS or specify in comments)
Atypical
• Endocervical cells, favor neoplastic
• Glandular cells, favor neoplastic
Endocervical adenocarcinoma in situ
Adenocarcinoma
• Endocervical
• Endometrial
• Extrauterine
• Not otherwise specified (NOS)

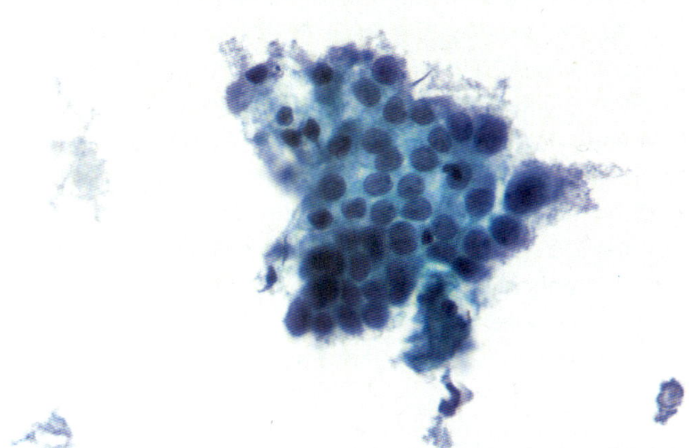

Fig. 2.5. Atypical endometrial cells. LBP. Serous endometrial adenocarcinoma. Pap, 40×.

with atypical squamous cells (ASC). The assessment 'favor reactive' has also been eliminated. The term 'atypical glandular cells' (AGC) gives the clinician more specific information.

– 'Atypical endocervical cells' and 'atypical glandular cells' may be qualified as 'favor neoplastic', but 'atypical endometrial cells' should not be further qualified. Current knowledge does not permit this subclassification.

– Atypical endometrial cells

Cytological Features. The cells occur in small three-dimensional groups with slight nuclear enlargement, mild hyperchromasia and inconspicuous nucleoli. Cell borders are poorly defined (fig. 2.4) [25]. In liquid-based preparations (LBP), nuclear hyperchromasia and nucleoli are usually more obvious [42]. It seems that liquid-based methods decrease the AGC rates but improve accuracy reducing the misinterpretation of squamous lesions as glandular [176] (fig. 2.5).

Assessment. In practice, a diagnosis of AGC is less frequently made than of ASC and has high interobserver variability. Atypical endometrial cells account for 5% of all AGC cases. One third of these have relevant uterine lesions, including endometrial polyps, hyperplasia and carcinoma. Other associated processes are chronic endometritis and IUD. The

The Value of Endometrial Cytology

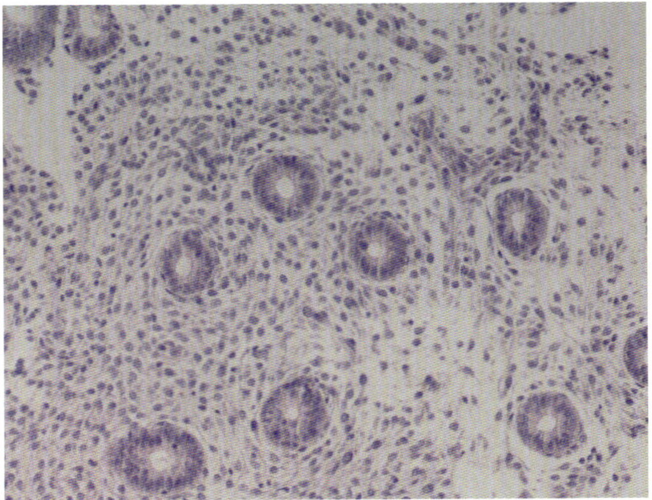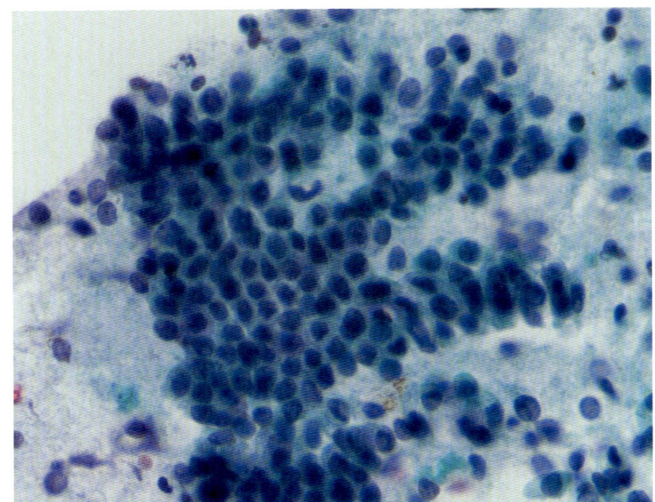

Fig. 2.6. Benign endometrial cells. **a** Cell block, HE, 20× and **b** Pap smear, 40×.

presence of cells with a nuclear size greater than twice that of intermediate cell nuclei, and the absence of clusters with irregular borders in an atrophic smear could be indicative of adenocarcinoma [177]. Endometrial lesions associated with AGC smears are unrelated to human papillomavirus infection [174].

Management. Consensus guidelines from the American Society for Colposcopy and Cervical Pathology (ASCCP) include recommendations for the initial workup and subsequent management of women with glandular abnormalities [226], based on the 2001 TBS [197]. Colposcopy and endocervical sampling are the suggested investigations of patients with adenocarcinoma in situ of endocervix (AIS) and AGC. Follow-up of AGC shows that high-grade lesions are found in 10–40% of cases, and are more often squamous cervical intraepithelial neoplasia 2 or 3 than glandular lesions. Endocervical sampling by brushing or curettage is recommended, as foci of high-grade squamous intraepithelial lesion and AIS may occur within the endocervical canal and be missed by colposcopy. Saad et al. [176] found significant uterine lesions in 40% of women who underwent biopsy following a diagnosis of AGC-endometrial cell. 82% were endometrial in origin, 18.2% were endometrial adenocarcinoma (EA) and 14.5% were endometrial hyperplasia (EH). Endometrial sampling is suggested in all patients with atypical endometrial cells, in those with AGC older than 35 years of age, and in those with abnormal vaginal bleeding regardless of age.

For women with AGC and no evidence of neoplasia in the initial workup, follow-up consists of a cervicovaginal smear (CVS) every 6 months, until 4 consecutive negative Paps are obtained. In cases of negative initial histological evaluation and persistent glandular atypia, the clinician should consider more aggressive investigation by a diagnostic excisional procedure (conization) [25, 30].

2.3. Benign Endometrial Cells in Cervicovaginal Smears

The reporting of endometrial cells found in CVS was revised in the Bethesda 2001 Conference. Many large studies have shown that women over 40 years of age may on some occasions present endometrial abnormalities, but that endometrial pathology is rare in women under 40. The rate of endometrial pathology increases after the age of 40. Cherkis et al. [29] noted an overall rate of 36% in this age group. Only 11% had an underlying carcinoma and most of these were elderly.

Unfortunately, when examining a Pap smear (Pap) the laboratory staff often has not received adequate clinical information or details of risk factors for endometrial carcinoma (EC) for the case. In view of the above facts, the conclusions of the 2001 TBS are that the presence of endometrial cells should only be reported in women 40 years of age or older.

Cytological Features. The exfoliated endometrial cells are found in ball-like clusters, the nuclei of which are of a similar size to intermediate cell nuclei with bland chromatin and inconspicuous nucleoli [173] (fig. 2.6). These nuclear features may be more clearly defined in LBP (fig. 2.7).

Assessment. For an adequate evaluation of benign endometrial cells, it is useful to take into consideration the following situations:

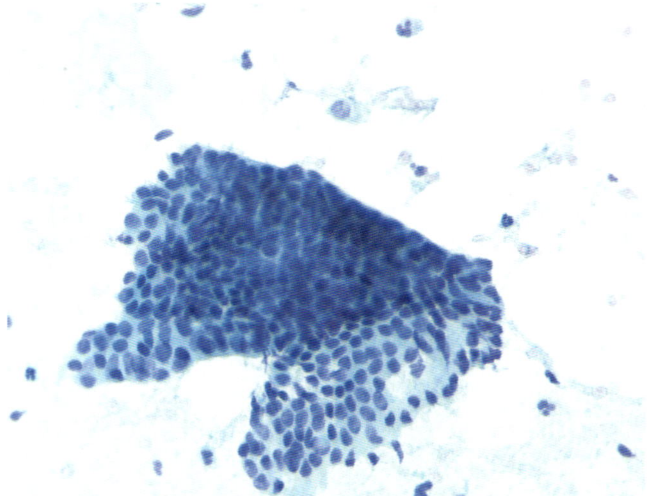

Fig. 2.7. Benign endometrial cells. LBP. Pap, 40×.

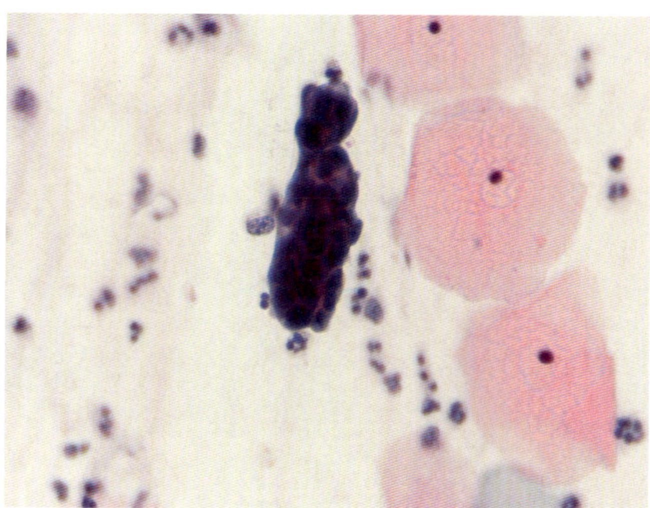

Fig. 2.8. Benign endometrial cells in an IUD user. Pap, 40×.

HRT in postmenopausal women: Some authors [139, 140] have found an increased prevalence of benign endometrial cells and endometrial disease in the Pap from postmenopausal women on HRT. However, these women have less abnormal endometrial histology than postmenopausal women who are not on HRT and who have benign endometrial cells in their CVS.

IUD: Users of an IUD can exfoliate benign endometrial cells until the 14th day of the normal cycle or later (fig. 2.8). It is important to inform the laboratory if the patient uses this type of contraceptive.

Instrumentation: Abraded endometrial cells of the lower uterine segment may be the result of a vigorous endocervical sampling (fig. 2.9) [138].

Educational Comment. The 2001 TBS suggests an optional comment when benign endometrial cells are found in a woman of 40 years or older. The endometrial cells have in most cases exfoliated from benign processes and only a small percentage of women have significant endometrial lesions [197]. The incidence ranged from 0 to 5% with a mean of 3%. Bean et al. [11] found that the incidence of EC in women over 40 was 0.47% before compared to 0.61% after implementation of the 2001 TBS, and that the difference was statistically significant. The incidence of clinically significant endometrial lesions associated with EM was very low, 1–4% and these patients were symptomatic. The authors recommend that women in this age group should have an endometrial biopsy only when additional clinical indicators are present [19]. These endometrial cells should be exfoliated glandular cells (not scraped, not histiocyte cells).

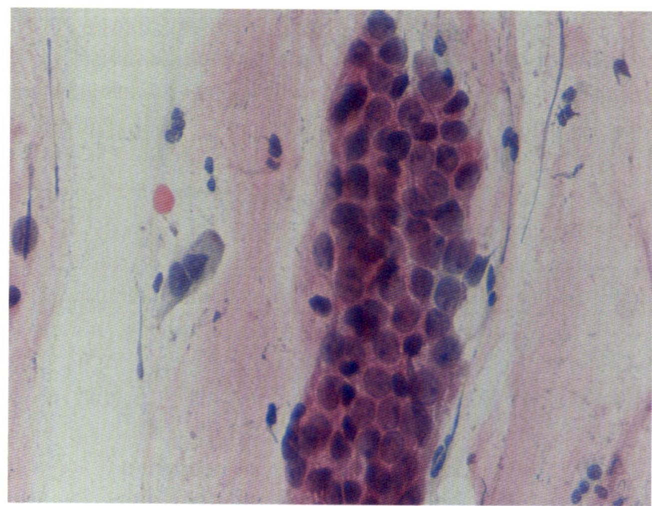

Fig. 2.9. Benign endometrial cells abraded from the LUS. Endocervical brushing. Pap, 60×.

2.4. Histiocytes and Psammoma Bodies

Histiocytes in association with exodus are frequently found in the postmenstrual Pap (fig. 2.10) [31, 138].

Isolated findings of histiocytes in the absence of postmenopausal bleeding, endometrial cells or AGC on a CVS smear have little relevance for endometrial pathology [147]. A significant clinical history is more important as an indicator for cytohistological study [221].

To complete our revision of some findings previously considered interesting, we would like to add that the presence of

The Value of Endometrial Cytology

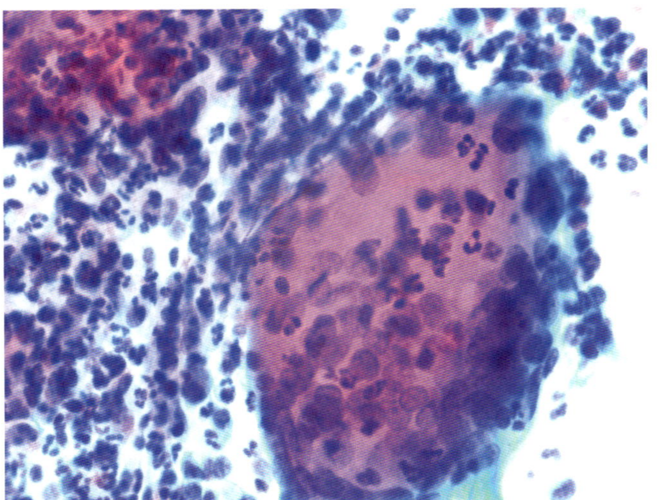

Fig. 2.10. Histiocytes in a Pap smear. 60×.

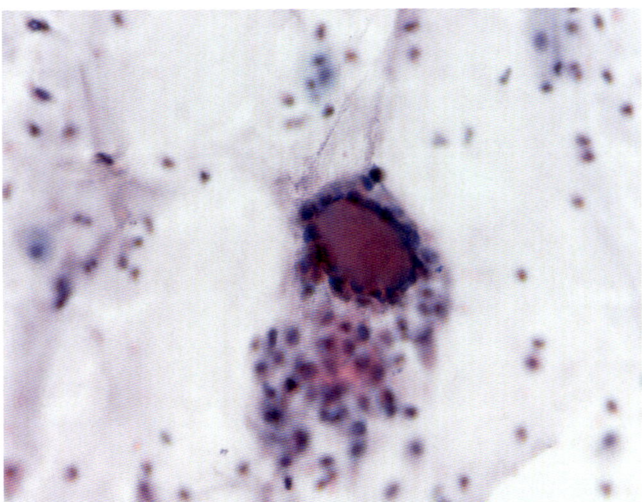

Fig. 2.11. Psammoma body in an endometrial carcinoma high grade. Pap, 60×.

psammoma bodies in normal smears (fig. 2.11) from asymptomatic women is now considered as an incidental finding [138].

2.5. Effectiveness of Endometrial Cytology in Detecting Endometrial Malignancy

Cervicovaginal Smear. The value of the information provided by the Pap with regard to endometrial pathology was summarized in the Conclusions of the Endometrial Forum of the 2001 Bethesda Conference: 'Cervical cytology is primarily a screening test for squamous cervical lesions, but is unsuitable for the detection of endometrial lesions' [197].

Conventionally the Pap is not expected to detect all endometrial neoplasias. As the sensitivity and specificity of CVS for the detection of this neoplasia are low, it is not a cost-effective screening tool for EC [111, 172]. It is estimated that among women who have an EA, only about one third shed abnormal cells that are detected in the Pap (fig. 2.12). The false-negative rate for EA of major studies varies between 55% [178] and 67% [106] or 68.7% [65].

Endometrial Brushing Techniques (EBT). Among the numerous techniques to obtain endometrial cytology samples, the best results have been achieved by EBT (fig. 2.13). The accuracy of EBT versus curettage and histological investigation has been tested using different instruments that we present in detail in Chapter 3. Most studies report satisfactory results in the detection of malignant lesions [196].

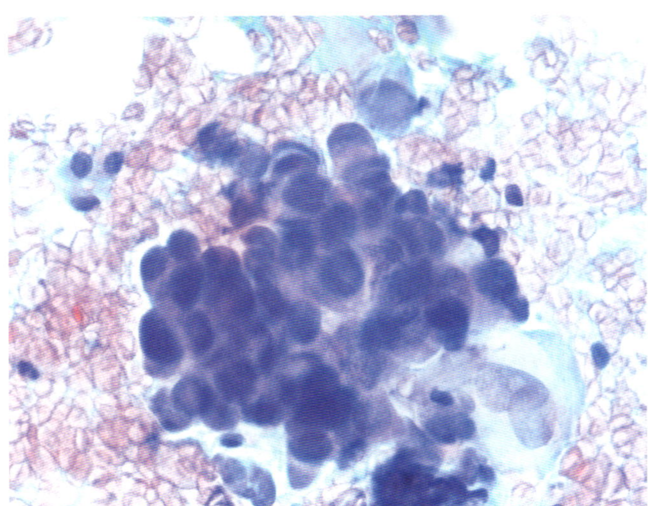

Fig. 2.12. Endometrial adenocarcinoma in Pap smear. 60×.

Adequacy of Samples. Criteria vary among investigators and with the type of endometrial lesions. An acceptable criterion for the diagnosis of non-malignant lesions is at least ten large fragments or clusters of endometrial epithelial cells. Five groups of well-preserved cancer cells are sufficient for the diagnosis of EC [150]. Correct sampling using the tested EBT yields relatively small numbers of malignant cells, 4–10% [150] and 4% [196].

Assessment of Endometrial Brushing Cytology. The specificity of EBT is high, ranging from 81 to 100% [150]. The

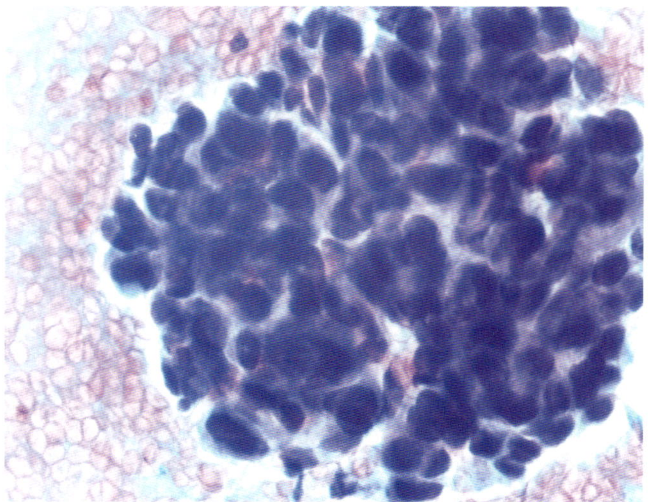

Fig. 2.13. Endometrial adenocarcinoma. Endometrial brushing by Medhosa cannula. Pap, 60×.

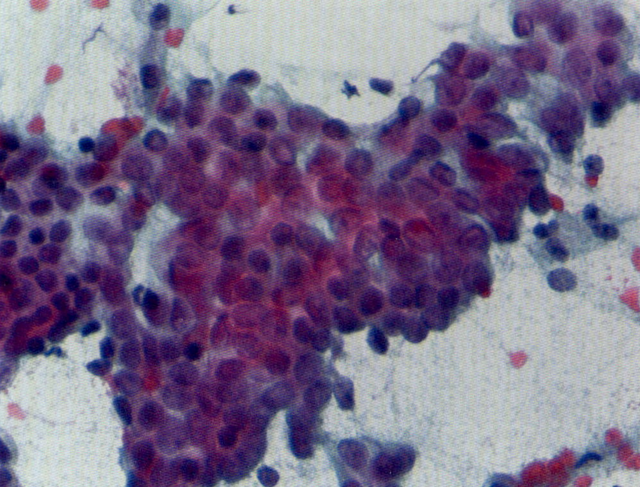

Fig. 2.14. Benign endometrial cells. LBP. Pap, 40×.

accuracy is higher for EC (Nguyen 93%, Skaarland no false-negatives). Tajima et al. [202] found 126 EC in 62,234 endometrial samples obtained by nylon brush. The false-positive rate was 8.7%, the positive predictive value was 85.7%, and the accuracy was 70% for EA. The accuracy is lower for EH (Nguyen 62%, Skaarland 10 of 50 cases). Kawawa et al. [104] found 11 cases among 687 cases of primary EC in which the neoplasia could be detected by endometrial aspiration cytology but not by endometrial curettage. They suppose that aspiration cytology may be a more sensitive diagnostic procedure than curettage for EC localized below the endometrial

surface and they confirm the usefulness of endometrial cytology in the early detection of cancer. In conclusion, to improve the accuracy of EBT, we must focus on the quality of sampling of material from premalignant lesions that make cytological evaluation difficult [196]. Most of the false-negative reports were due to insufficient material, pale staining in malignant cells or diagnostic error [202].

Endometrial Brushing Techniques and Liquid-Based Cytology. An update of the value of endometrial cytology using both techniques will be presented in Chapter 3 (fig. 2.14).

The Value of Endometrial Cytology

Techniques of Endometrial Cytology

3.1. Techniques for the Detection and Early Diagnosis of Endometrial Cancer

The current techniques for the detection and early diagnosis of endometrial cancer (EC) can be divided into three groups:

Cytology: The cytological techniques are presented in this chapter.

Histopathology: Endometrial tissue for histology can be taken as an office procedure (Pipelle, microbiopsies) or by an endometrial curettage (D&C). These techniques will be described in Chapter 4 [196].

Other Gynecological Techniques: Transvaginal sonography is the imaging technique of choice for the assessment of the endometrium in symptomatic patients. The value of this technique and of hysteroscopy will be discussed by Dr. E. Iglesias and Dr. M. Rios in Chapter 5. Magnetic resonance imaging has no established role in the screening for EC but it is the best technique for preoperative staging and is superior to computed tomography.

3.2. Techniques of Endometrial Cytology

For a cytological technique to be accepted as a useful tool for endometrial screening it must first be proven to be an inexpensive, simple (can be used by any gynecologist) and painless sampling method that is able to obtain representative endometrial cells. Secondly, it must be shown that accurate interpretation of samples is possible [165]. Special experience is needed to screen endometrial smears. Cell morphology and diagnostic criteria are different from those of Pap smears (Pap). One common difficulty is the differentiation between endometrial and endocervical cells in cases of glandular pathology [129].

Endometrial Aspiration Techniques. After Papanicolaou's publication [167] of the Cannule of Cary, many types of cannulas have been proposed to obtain endometrial specimens by aspiration procedures. The use of all of these has been long discontinued, mainly due to the risk of spreading malignant cells. Vassilakos et al. [215] used a metallic or polyethylene cannula. The Isaac endometrial cell sampler (fig. 3.1) has a metallic cannula and a specimen collector [216]. Bibbo [15] reported good results with a 'vakutage' device, and Jensen and Jensen [87] introduced the Vabra aspiration. The disadvantages of the last three aspiration procedures are lack of simplicity and high cost.

Endometrial Brushing Techniques (EBT). One important advantage of these techniques is that samples are processed similarly to other gynecologic specimens using the standard Papanicolaou staining technique. Among the different techniques for obtaining endometrial cytology samples, the commonest are EBT [49, 159, 229], which we prefer ourselves. We have ample experience with Medhosa, Mi-Mark, Endobrush and Endopap methods. The EBT are reviewed and re-evaluated in the following section [93, 94, 100].

3.2.1. The Medhosa Cannula

We were the first to use this device [90, 91]. The Medhosa endometrial brushing cannula (fig. 3.2) is 30 cm long, made of plastic and is slightly curved to facilitate entry into the cervical canal and uterine cavity without danger of perforation.

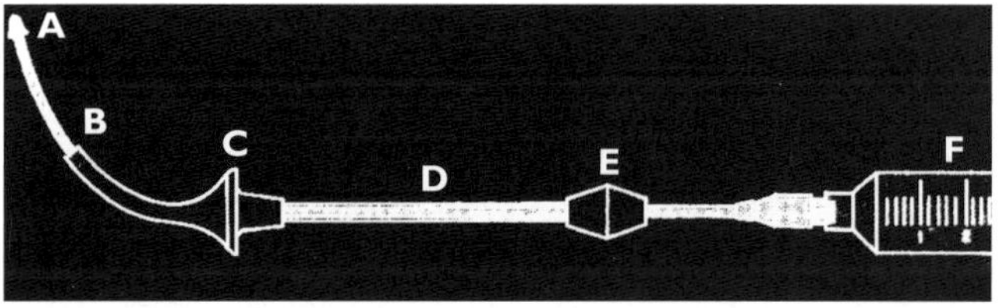

Fig. 3.1. Isaac endometrial sampler.

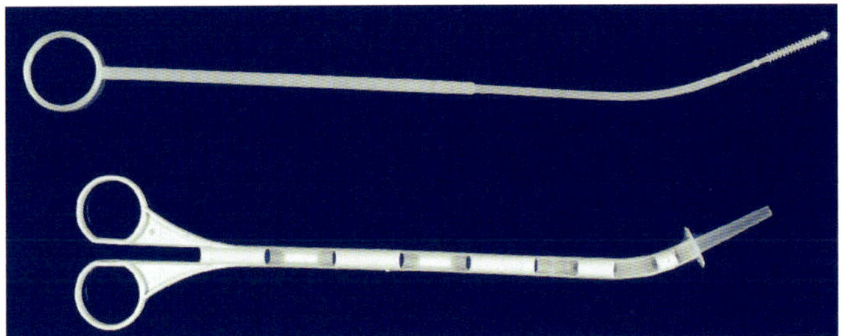

Fig. 3.2. Medhosa endometrial brushing cannula.

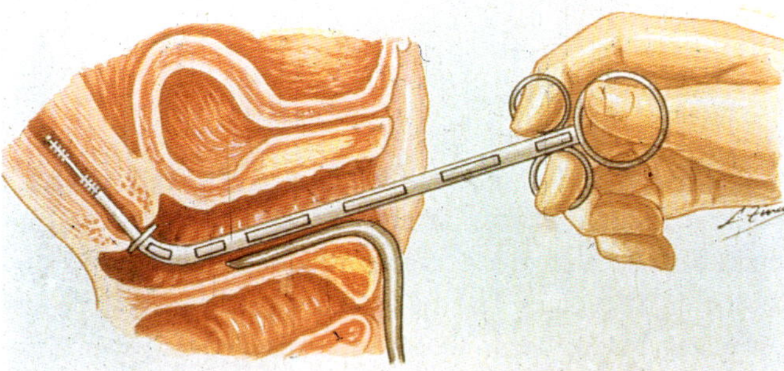

Fig. 3.3. Endometrial sample taken with Medhosa's cannula.

It has a guide and a plunger. The guide has an introduction cone at the end equipped with a stop to avoid penetration when it hits the cervix. The plunger has thin, flexible fins designed to sweep or brush the endometrium.

Endometrial samples are taken as follows (fig. 3.3): The introduction cone is inserted into the endocervical canal; the cone of the cannula houses the thinnest part of the piston so that it will not touch the cervix. Once the endometrial brushing is completed, the piston is removed and the material is spread on a slide [92].

Table 3.1 lists the advantages of the EBT by the Medhosa cannula. There are practically no inconveniences.

In 1995 (J. Ayala, Goldblatt Lecture) we conducted an enquiry in 24 Spanish hospitals on the results of available EBT. The largest number of cases (n = 98,481) was by the Medhosa cannula. No endometrial material was obtained in 6.78%. 1,086 EA were diagnosed. There were 5.13% false-positive and 3.97% false-negative reports (table 3.2) [92].

3.2.2. Mi-Mark Helix Technique

The Mi-Mark endometrial sampling kit contains two disposable plastic instruments (fig. 3.4). The helix has semisharp edges to abrade the endometrial lining and it is associated with a thin probe to dilate the cervix. After its insertion into the uterus, the helix takes the endometrial material by a rotational 'screwing' movement. Any remaining material is fixed for histological processing [44, 125].

Table 3.1. Endometrial cytodiagnosis: Medhosa's cannula brushing

Advantages
Painless, good patient acceptance. Suitable for ambulatory sampling. Simple and quick. Cervix clamps, cervix dilation, analgesia, anesthesia all unnecessary
Absence of complications such as perforation, bleeding, infection
Sterilized presentation
Abundant and well-preserved material. High level of diagnostic accuracy

Inconveniences
Low incidence of insufficient cytological material

Table 3.2. Endometrial cytodiagnosis: Medhosa's cannula brushing

Cases	Inadequate	Correlation cyt./hist.	Adenoc.	False-positives	False-negatives
98,491	6.78%	22.67%	1,086	5.13%	3.97%

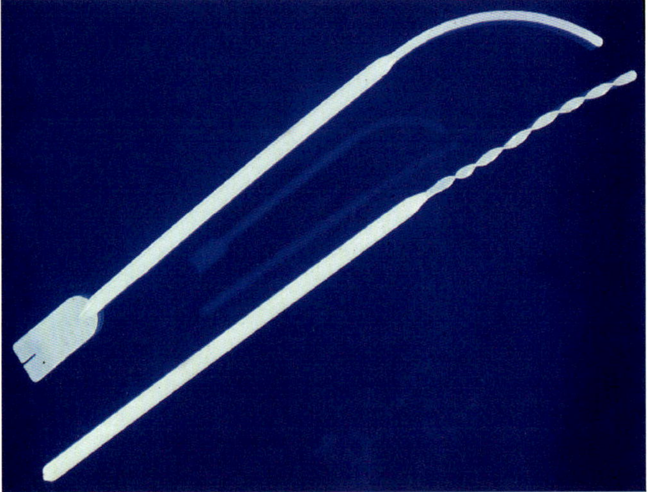

Fig. 3.4. Mi-Mark endometrial sampling kit.

Results of the Technique
Adequacy. Most authors obtained satisfactory and adequate endometrial material for diagnosis (Cramer in 96% of 170 cases) [43]. Crow et al. [44] reported 30% of inadequate material in smears from a series of 115 patients. In our review of the results from 9 Spanish institutions including 85,707 patients, 8.23% of samples had insufficient material [92]. Uvebrant et al. [211] found that Mi-Mark specimens from a series of 736 patients had inadequate material for

Techniques of Endometrial Cytology

Author	Cases	Inadequate (%)	Correlation cyt./hist. (%)	Adenoc.	False-positives (%)	False-negatives (%)	Sensitivity (%)	Specificity (%)
Spanish hospitals	85,707	8.23	26.31	712	8.61	2.47		
Cramer	170	4.0		9			97	96
Crow	115	30		3				
Urebrant	736	11–30						
Burati	335	15.6		14			93	

diagnosis in 11% of the premenopausal and in 30% of the postmenopausal women. For this reason, the Mi-Mark helix is not recommended in the older age group. Buratti et al. [23] found that in a series of 335 women at risk of EC, endometrial material could not be obtained with the Mi-Mark helix in 5.6% of cases, and that the endometrial samples were inadequate for diagnosis in another 10% (table 3.3).

Accuracy. Cramer and Osborne [43] found a sensitivity of 97%, a specificity of 96% and a predictive value for EA of 97%, with 9 cases of EA. In Buratti's series of 335 women, the sensitivity for EA was 93%, the sensitivity for atypical hyperplasia (AH) was 62%, and that for hyperplasia without atypia was 76% [23]. Markley and Milan [134] reported 90% sensitivity for EA. In our review of the Spanish institutions [92], there were 712 cases of EA with 8.61% false-positives and 2.4% false-negatives. Most of the authors concluded that the Milan-Markley helix is satisfactory technique.

3.2.3. Endobrush

The Endobrush device for EBT is composed of a plastic tube or guide, 2.5 mm in diameter, and a helicoidal thin wire with a nylon brush, with a plastic enlargement on the end (fig. 3.5). The Endobrush is inserted through the cervical canal up to the fundus. The uterine cavity is brushed after the tube has been withdrawn.

Results of Technique. The results of EBT by Endobrush are acceptable. Vuopala et al. [217] obtained adequate samples in 94% of 113 cases, and Methelin et al. [124] in 74% of 189 patients treated with tamoxifen. The rate of inadequate samples is low; Vuopala 2.8%, the Spanish institutions 9.79% in 12,039 cases. However, Methelin reported 28% inadequate samples in postmenopausal breast cancer patients.

Accuracy. Vuopala did not have any false-negative findings in 113 cases, but the number of EA was only 5 and there were 2 false-positives. His findings in EH were unsatisfactory. Methelin did not have any false-negatives but overestimated the risk of endometrial pathology in 5 patients, 1 of whom was given a diagnosis of cancer [123, 124]. In a review of figures

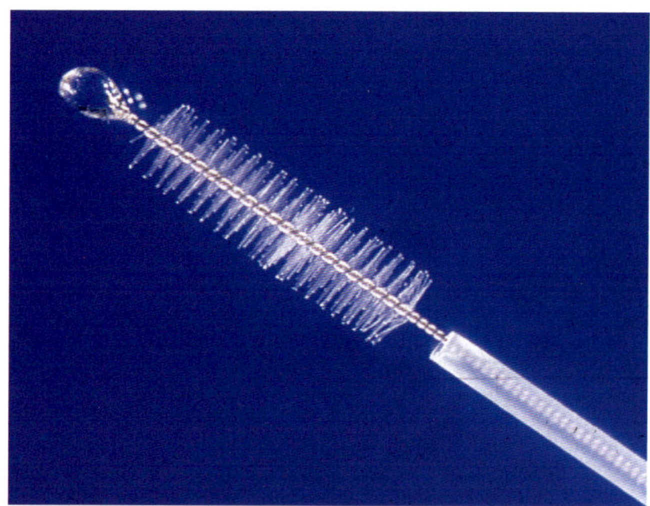

Fig. 3.5. Endobrush device for endometrial brushing techniques.

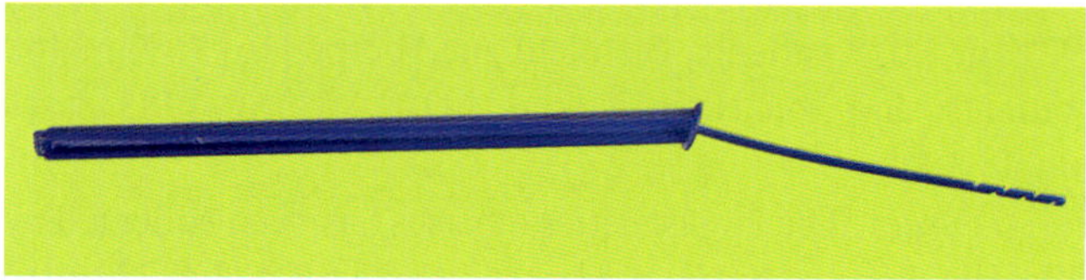

Fig. 3.6. Endopap device for endometrial brushing.

from four Spanish hospitals, we found 178 cases of EA with 2.16% false-positive diagnoses and 6% false-negatives [92].

In conclusion, the Endobrush endometrial device seems to be a simple, quick and painless method with acceptable results.

3.2.4. Endopap

Introduced by Palermo [165], the device consists of a piece of soft plastic with a 2-mm thick dart and 6 small cavities, through which the endouterine brushing is performed (fig. 3.6).

Table 3.4. Endometrial cytodiagnosis: Endopap brushing

Author	Cases	Inadequate (%)	Adenoc.	Sensitivity (%)	Specificity (%)	Sensitive hyperplasias (%)
Meisels	9,710	21.72	68	85	96.9	45.5
Palermo	1,027	8	36		94	31
Bistoletti	468	4	134		96	97–90
Van Hoeven	1,983	15	4		95	
Whitaker				95		69.2
Van den Bosch		10.6	5	80		
La Polla		2.49		90		58

Table 3.5. Cytopathology of the uterus (Meisels): endometrial cytology by direct sampling over a 15-year period

Cytology	Case load	
	n	%
Benign	7,294	75.12
Atypical	232	2.37
Malignant	75	0.77
Inadequate	2,109	21.72
Total	9,710	99.98[1]

[1]Total does not equal 100% because of rounding.

Table 3.6. Cytopathology of the uterus (Meisels): comparison of histology and cytology in 1,825 women

Histology	Cytology			
	benign	atypical	malignant	total
Benign	1,426	48	8	1,482
Simple hyperplasia	229	9	4	242
Atypical hyperplasia	16	6	1	23
Malignant	13	8	57	78
Total	1,684	71	701	1,825

Results of Technique

Adequacy. The diagnostic adequacy of samples obtained by EBT by Endopap is acceptable; Meisels and Morin [131] reported 78.28% adequacy in 9,710 cases, Palermo [165] 92% in 1,027 patients, Bistoletti and Hjerpe [16] 96% in 468 patients, and Van Hoeven et al. [214] 85% in 1983 cases (table 3.4).

Accuracy. The largest series of cases has been collected by Meisels. His results are presented in tables 3.4–3.6. Thirteen of 78 malignant tumors were missed by cytology (sensitivity 85%) and 56 of 1,482 benign cases were reported as atypical [48] or malignant [8] (specificity 96.9%). Palermo obtained a specificity of 94% in 36 cases of EA, and Bistoletti and Hjerpe [16] a specificity of 96% in 134 EA. Whitaker and Knight [222] found a sensitivity of 95%, Van den Bosch et al. [213] 80%, and La Polla et al. [116] 90%. Finally, van Hoeven et al. [214] reported a specificity of 95% in 1,983 cases but the overall sensitivity for all pathologic lesions was only 28%.

The accuracy of the cytodiagnosis of EH is lower than of endometrial neoplasia; Whitaker reported 69.2% sensitivity, La Polla 58%, Meisels 45.5% and Palermo 31%, but Bistoletti and Hjerpe found a specificity of 97% in AH and of 90% in EH without atypia.

Palermo regards the Endopap sampler as a minicurette that collects the material in a way similar to a curettage. Its extended use reduces the number of fractional curettages [165].

In conclusion, it is accepted that the Endopap is a simple and economical method, which has proven to be effective in detecting EA, but which is not reliable in the diagnosis of EH. Special training is necessary in cytological diagnosis.

3.3. Spanish Endometrial Experience

The Spanish cytologist M. de Arcos [4] named the Spanish School of Endometrial Cytology having found that over a long time Spanish cytopathologists have accumulated a wide experience resulting in uniformity of criteria in endometrial cytology. Spanish cytopathologists have used generally accepted endometrial brushing devices, and their experience has been documented in several multicentric studies (Paris 1976, Barcelona 1982, Montreal 1983). The Spanish experience up to 1995 including a total of 219,449 patients was reviewed in a survey from 24 Spanish hospitals

Table 3.7. Endometrial cytodiagnosis (Jiménez-Ayala, 1995)

Techniques	Cases	Inadequate (%)	Correlation cyt./hist.	%	Adenoc.	False-positives (%)	False-negatives (%)
Medhosa[1]	3,331	3.27	763	22.91	78	7.35	1.49
Endobrush[1]	404	3.00	159	39.35	7	0	0
Mi-Mark	8,298	12.13	1,880	22.66	110	3.22	1.50
Total	12,033	6.13	2,802	28.30	195	3.52	1.00

[1]Plus Vilaplana.

Table 3.8. Technical evaluation of endometrial sampling

Technique	Difficulties	Complications	Pros	Cons	Sample quality	Comments
Medhosa	Few (in penetration, cervical stenosis)	None	Simplicity	None	Good	Satisfactory
Mi-Mark	Few	None	Endocervical screening	Pain	Good	Satisfactory
Endobrush	Few	None	Simplicity	None	Acceptable	Just acceptable
Endopap	Few	None	Almost painless	Unavailable	Good	Satisfactory
Cornier	Few	None	For endometrial biopsy	Poor samples	High percentage of inadequacy	Acceptable for outpatient biopsy; unsuitable for cytology

and reported by us in the Goldblatt Award Lecture of the XII International Congress of Cytology in Madrid, May 1995. We found that 1,086 of EA had been diagnosed with 5.13% false-positive and 3.9% false-negative reports [92]. I also presented our personal experience of 12,033 cases over 24 years using EBT with Medhosa, Endobrush and Mi-Mark devices (table 3.7). In summary, the material was inadequate in 6.13%. 195 EA were diagnosed with 3.52% false-positives and 1.00% false-negatives [92]. Finally, our technical evaluation of endometrial sampling by the devices used by Spanish cytopathologists is summarized in table 3.8.

3.4. Tao Brush

The Tao endometrial sampler, introduced in 1993 in Indiana University Medical Center, is a long brush with a 16-cm outer protection, similar to an Endobrush, and employing

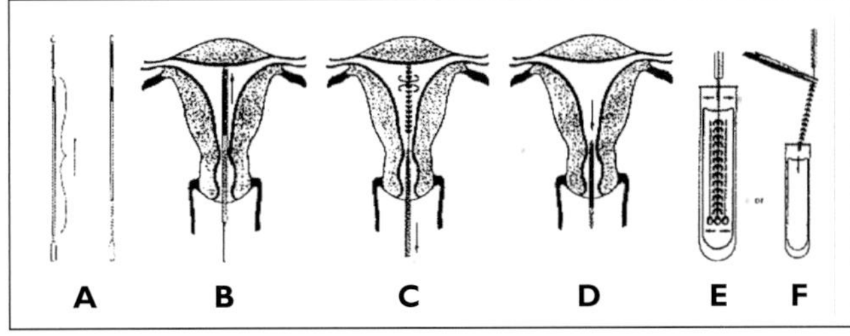

Fig. 3.7. Tao endometrial brush.

the same procedure of endometrial sampling (fig. 3.7). The processing of material is not simple: it needs the centrifugation of samples in suspension and the use of special fixatives. Wu et al. [227] and Maksem [121] have reported a technical modification which allows histological examination.

Results of Technique. The adequacy of endometrial samples is variable. Maksem obtained 30% inadequate samples

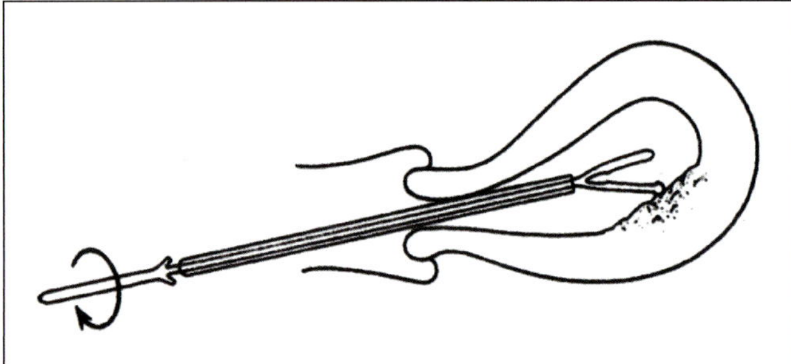

Fig. 3.8. Endocyte endometrial brush.

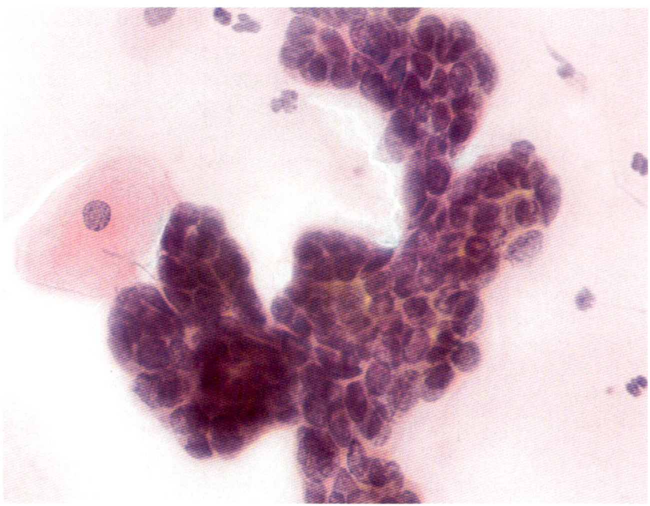

Fig. 3.9. Liquid-based cytology: metastatic cancer of ovary. Pap, 60×.

in 50 cases, but Wu obtained 90% satisfactory endometrial brush samples in 633 cases.

Accuracy. The reported accuracy for this technique is acceptable. Wu found a sensitivity in AH of 89% and in EC of 96%. Smith et al. [196] found a sensitivity of endometrial cytology for detecting EH/EA of 57% and a specificity of 98%.

Currently, the Tao brush endometrial technique can be considered as an accurate and safe, but not simple procedure to be used in the outpatients setting to study endometrial pathology. Wu stated that it has the advantage over the Pipelle biopsy of being well tolerated by patients. A detailed description and results with the endometrial pathological device Pipelle is presented in the Chapter 4. We feel that the Tao brush does not meet all the requirements for use in the initial evaluation of women at high risk for EC.

3.5. Other Endometrial Techniques

Endocyte

Device. The Endocyte is a two-piece flexible plastic disposable device of 216 × 2.6 mm. The outer section is a protective plastic tube and the inner polypropylene sampler scrapes the endometrial epithelium (fig. 3.8). It resembles an IUD, and is easy to use by gynecologists [203].

Results of Technique. The adequacy of endometrial material obtained by Endocyte is acceptable. In Byrne's [24] series of 874 patients, 8.2% of the samples were inadequate for diagnosis. The inadequate rate was 8% in Ferency and Gelfand's [61] 200 cases (table 3.9).

Accuracy. The reported accuracy of the Endocyte has been satisfactory. Byrne found that cytology had a sensitivity of 92% and a specificity of 100% for the diagnosis of benign versus malignant lesions. Ferency and Gelfand confirmed the cytological diagnosis of EH in 80.5% and of EC in 100% in a series of 200 cases. 19.5% of hyperplasias were underdiagnosed as normal endometrium. Porrazzi [41, 169] found a sensitivity of 81% and a specificity and positive predictive value of 100% in 1,248 asymptomatic women. The sensitivity was 96%, the specificity 98% and the positive predictive value 75% in 550 symptomatic women. Zarcone et al. [233] found 96.55% of diagnostic concordance in 145 endometrial cytologic samples.

In conclusion, the Endocyte method is inexpensive, easy to use by a gynecologist and is well tolerated by patients. It seems to be useful for screening asymptomatic woman at risk of EC but histology is preferable in symptomatic patients [169].

Endoscan. Several devices similar to Endocyte have been introduced. The Endoscan consists of a flexible plastic tube and a curved rod. Segadal [182] reported adequate material in 92% of 200 patients, and diagnostic agreement in 21 of 23 EC and in 2 of 5 cases with premalignant disease.

Endosearch. This method was developed in Japan by Noda [153]. It consists of an inner shaft and an external tube that also collects endometrial tissue in 88.5% of 78 cases. Cytologic endometrial material was satisfactory in 98.9% of cases [210]. The reported accuracy of the results is acceptable.

Softcyte. This is another disposable polypropylene instrument like the Endocyte. The success in getting endometrial specimens is about 90–95%. Nagai et al. [144] reported good results in 315 patients.

3.6. New Resources for Endometrial Cytologic Diagnosis

Liquid-Based Cytology (LBP). LBP is a new method of collecting and preparing cell samples. These are obtained

Techniques of Endometrial Cytology

Table 3.9. Endometrial cytodiagnosis: Endocyte brushing

Author	Cases	Inadequate (%)	Adenoc.	Sensitivity (%)	Specificity (%)	Spec. hyperplasia (%)
Byrne	874	8.2		92	100	
Ferency	200	8			10	80.5
Porrazzi	1,248		28	81	100	
	550			96	98	
Zarcone	145			96.55		

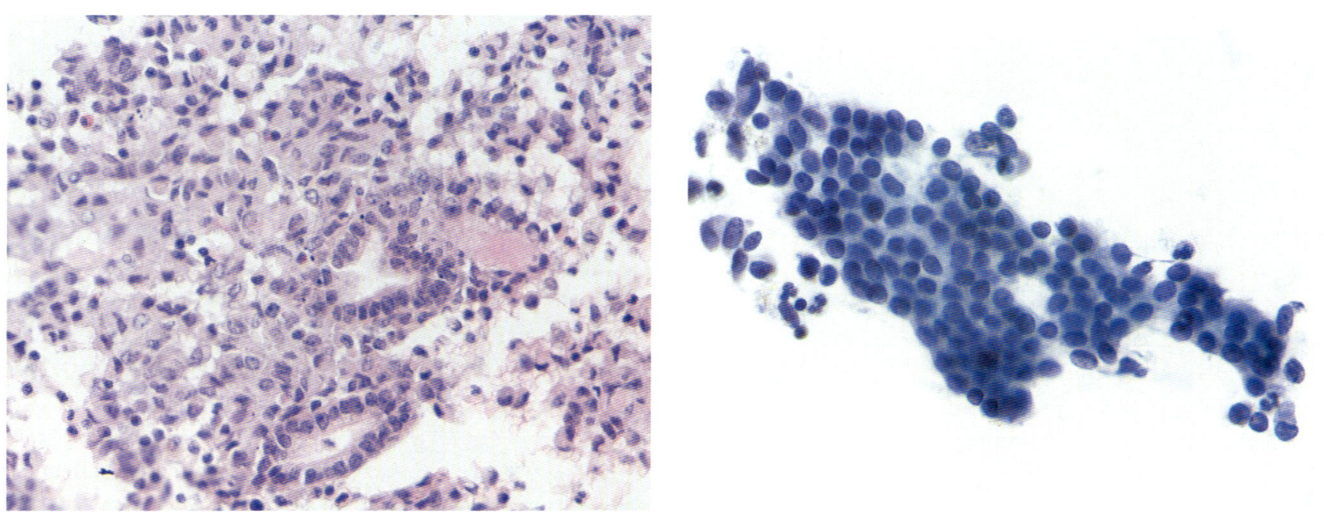

Fig. 3.10. Proliferative endometrium with glandular and stromal breakdown. **a** Cell block: HE, 20×, and **b** LBP: Pap, 40×.

using different devices, most commonly brushing techniques for endometrial cytology. The material is placed into a vial with methanol or an ethanol-based preservative/fixative, and sent to the Laboratory. The sample is then processed and deposited on a slide as a thin layer of cells. The LBP includes automated and semiautomated techniques and preparations by cytocentrifugation. The ThinPrep (TP) Pap Test (Cytyc Corp.), and the SurePath LBC (TricPath Imaging, Inc.) are the two LBPs approved by the US Food and Drug Administration. Both methods are relatively expensive procedures [131].

Cells in LBP will appear smaller than in conventional smears since they are fixed in their three-dimensional state. Glandular cells may 'round up' into balls making interpretation more problematic. This difficulty is reduced by focusing on different planes at edges of such cell clusters. Parabasal cells can be misinterpreted as endometrial cells [131].

Published reports refer to greater difficulty in recognizing glandular lesions, decreased sensitivity for EA, or increased detection of cervical and endometrial glandular lesions [8, 48, 72]. Ashfag et al. [6] found similar overall rates of glandular cytology for conventional smears, 0.11% of 43,284 smears and TP cytology 0.14% of 25,783 slides. A statistically significant reduction in the false-negative rate was noted with the TP method (1 vs. 4 cases; p < 0.2). TP has proven to be more sensitive in detecting EA (65.2 vs. 38.6% by conventional cytology; p = 0.010) [181]. Papaefthimiou et al. [166] has used TP with an Endogyn endometrial device in 491 postmenopausal women and found a sensitivity of 98.08% specificity of 100%, positive predictive value of 100%, negative predictive value of 100% and overall accuracy of 98.98%. However, unfortunately this is a high cost and complex method (fig. 3.9).

Cell Block Preparation. Diaz-Rosario and Kabawat [52] devised a novel technique to prepare cell blocks that avoids disruption of glandular structure during preparation. The fluid remaining after the preparation of the TP slide is subjected to sedimentation in the inverted TP filter cylinder used for slide preparation. Sediment is separated from the filter at the bottom of the cylinder. Filter and sediment are processed for histology as a cell block. The authors and Kyroudi et al. [113] found that the inverted filter sedimentation is useful in the differential diagnosis of AGC. Kyroudi used the histological material obtained by inverted filter cylinder and the cytological material obtained by TP for diagnosis which increased the diagnostic accuracy of endometrial cytology to 96.3% for benign/atrophic endometrium, to 100% for EA, to 96% for EH without atypia, and to 95.3% for AH. Direct endometrial smears are much easier and faster to prepare than cell blocks, but more difficult to interpret [113, 114]. The interpretation of the tissue patterns in cell blocks or microbiopsies is much easier, although the preparation is tissue consuming [107] (fig. 3.10a, b).

Autopath 300. Autopath 300, approved for primary screening of conventional cervical smears, is slightly less sensitive than manual screening by an experienced cytotechnologist, for the detection of endometrial cells in conventional smears. For most patients, routine use of primary screening of conventional smears is unlikely to contribute to delays in the diagnosis of clinically significant endometrial lesions [218].

Techniques of Endometrial Cytology

Chapter 4

Techniques of Endometrial Histopathology

Many gynecological consultations, especially those related to abnormal vaginal bleeding, warrant study of the endometrium. Traditionally the standard method of assessing the endometrium has been dilatation of the cervix and curettage (D&C) of the uterine cavity under general anesthesia. Lately, simple, quick, safe and inexpensive methods have superseded D&C. Cytological techniques have been described in Chapter 3 and in the current chapter we will describe the techniques to obtain material for histological study. Endometrial tissue for histology can be taken as an office procedure, D&C or by hysteroscopy and curettage (tables 4.1, 4.2)

4.1. Office Procedures (tables 4.3, 4.4)

4.1.1. Vacuum-Based Sampling Techniques

These are the most popular endometrial sampling devices. Material is obtained by suction generated in one of three ways: internal piston, vacuum syringe or vacuum pump.

Results of the Technique

The failure rate of aspiration techniques is approximately 10%, the proportion of inadequate samples is 13% and 5% of women report substantial pain. Regarding diagnostic accuracy, aspiration techniques (Pipelle, Vabra, Vakutage), compared to scraping, lavage or a combination, give the best performance in detecting hyperplasia and endometrial carcinoma. However, there is evidence that supports the contention that malignant pathology can be missed by outpatient biopsy and, therefore, additional endometrial assessment should be undertaken if the material is insufficient, if symptoms persist or if intrauterine structural abnormalities are suspected. In that case, hysteroscopy and curettage are recommended [21].

Table 4.1. Techniques to obtain material for histological study

4.1. Office procedures
    4.1.1. Vacuum-based sampling techniques
        4.1.1.1. Internal piston
        Pipelle
        Z-sampler
        Gynosampler
        4.1.1.2. Vacuum syringe
        Novak curette
        Accurette
        Uterine Explora curette
        4.1.1.3. Vacuum pump (electric suction devices)
        Vabra aspirator
        Masterson endometrial biopsy system
        Tis-U-Trap
    4.1.2. Brushing technique
    Mimark helix
4.2. Dilatation & curettage
4.3. Hysteroscopy and curettage

Table 4.2. Indications of endometrial sampling

– Evaluate abnormal uterine bleeding
– Diagnose endometrial cancer or hyperplasia
– Monitor the effects of hormone replacement therapy
– Determine the potential causes of infertility

Table 4.3. Advantages of office procedures

– More convenient for patient and physician
– Generally does not require cervical dilatation
– Anesthesia or analgesia optional, depending on patient's needs
– Lower rate of complications (uterine haemorrhage, infection and perforation)
– Approximately 1/10 the cost of D&C per procedure

Table 4.4. Disadvantages of office procedures

– Blind procedure
– Small false-negative rate. Negative results, including inadequate sampling, must be interpreted with caution
– Possible errors in histological typing and grading of neoplasia

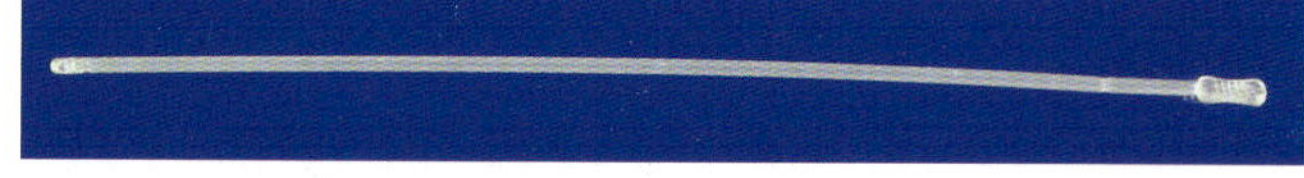

Fig. 4.1. Internal piston device 'Pipelle de Cornier-like'.

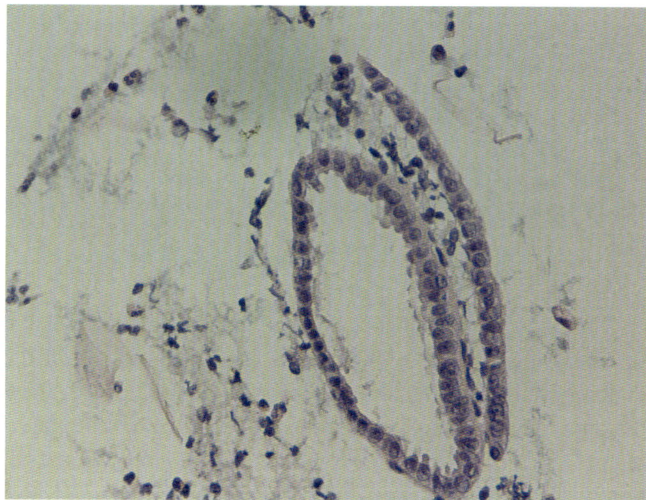

Fig. 4.2. 'Scanty non-diagnostic material, further investigation recommended'.

4.1.1.1. Internal Piston

Internal piston devices generate suction that draws a column of tissue into the tube when the piston is pulled back (fig. 4.1).

Pipelle

The Pipelle de Cornier was described in 1984 [39]. It is made of flexible plastic and is 23.5 cm in length and has a 3.1-mm external diameter with a distal circular port. After the device is inserted into the uterine cavity, negative pressure is generated by pulling back an internal piston. A specimen is then obtained by simultaneously rotating and moving the device in and out several times within the uterine cavity. After the Pipelle is withdrawn from the uterus, the distal tip is removed and the specimen is expelled by advancing the piston. Innovative features of the Pipelle as compared to previous devices were the soft plastic tip, the somewhat smaller distal opening and the plunger or 'piston' by which the suction is applied. The cannula is its own collecting chamber and the instrument was disposable, which was a commercial innovation as well.

Results of the Technique

The Pipelle is the most extensively studied 'office' sampler. Several studies have compared it with the Vabra aspirator, Novak curette, Tis-U-Trap [105], Accurette and Explora [120], etc. The Pipelle is equal to or better than these samplers as regards the yield of tissue for histological analysis and patient comfort.

In a meta-analysis comparing the results of several office endometrial sampling techniques with D&C, hysteroscopy, and/or hysterectomy, the authors found that the Pipelle device was superior to other techniques of endometrial sampling in the detection of endometrial carcinoma and atypical hyperplasia, especially in postmenopausal women [54]. In both post- and premenopausal women, the Pipelle was the best device for the detection of endometrial carcinoma, with a sensitivity of 99.6 and 91%, respectively. For the detection of atypical hyperplasia, the Pipelle device was the most sensitive technique, with a sensitivity of 81%. Endometrial biopsy taken with the Pipelle is highly accurate when the diagnosis is positive. However, if the findings are negative, the material may not be representative and other outpatient methods such as vaginal sonography or outpatient hysteroscopy should be performed before scheduling conventional curettage, particularly in patients with risk factors (fig. 4.2) [122]. Another possible disadvantage of the Pipelle is that the initial typing and grading of endometrial carcinomas made on the Pipelle sample may not agree with the final diagnosis obtained after hysterectomy (fig. 4.3) [179].

Other Internal Piston Devices

Some devices similar to the Pipelle de Cornier have been described, like the Z-sampler [118] and the Gynosampler. The principal difference between the Gynosampler and the Pipelle is the greater degree of rigidity or stiffness of the former. The Gynosampler is comparable to Pipelle in terms of adequacy of samples of endometrial tissue obtained and the degree of patient discomfort associated with the biopsy procedure. However, the Gynosampler is easier to use than the Pipelle [136].

4.1.1.2. Vacuum Syringe
Novak Curette

In 1935, Novak [157] introduced the first instrument designed specifically for in-office endometrial biopsy.

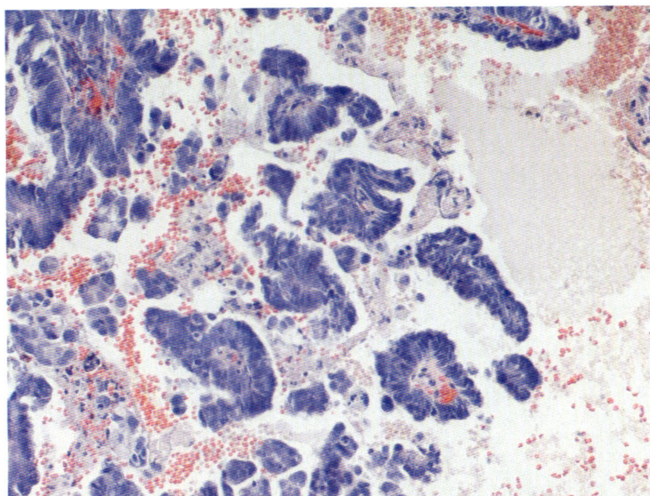

Fig. 4.3. A papillary carcinoma may be suspected, but the diagnosis obtained after hysterectomy was an endometrioid carcinoma with focal papillary areas.

Despite the subsequent introduction and evaluation of several other devices designed specifically for in-office endometrial biopsy over the past 70 years, the Novak curette has remained relatively unchanged in design and has been the endometrial biopsy instrument to which most new devices have been compared.

The Novak curette is a rigid, stainless steel, non-disposable cannula with a 4.2-mm outer diameter and a 3.2-mm inner diameter, measuring 25 cm in length with a blunt rounded tip. There is a serrated 1-cm long by 3.2-mm wide opening 3 mm from the distal end. When negative pressure is applied to the instrument by a syringe attached to the proximal end, endometrial contents are drawn into the cannula and syringe [118].

Results of the Technique

Some studies have compared the Novak curette and the Pipelle, finding similar adequacy and quality in the samples. However, the Novak curette is associated with a greater amount of pain than the flexible plastic alternatives.

Other Devices with Vacuum Syringe

Accurette: This device was proposed in 1982 for obtaining samples of the endometrium for both cytology and histology. It consists of a disposable, collapsible curette made from a special plastic material with a simple syringe attached for vacuum aspiration.

A sample of the endometrium is removed by scraping and collected into a syringe [108]. Although a good diagnostic accuracy was reported in the first studies [198], later studies did not recommend the Accurette for endometrial sampling. Lipscomb et al. [120] recorded a 42% unsatisfactory rate and Spicer et al. [199] obtained an inadequate histological diagnosis in 65 of 136 samples in a prospective study performed on 102 consecutive patients with postmenopausal bleeding.

Uterine Explora Curette

The uterine Explora curette is a flexible 3-mm nylon curette with a Randall-type cutting edge obturator. A 12-cc Vacu-Lok syringe is used to provide negative pressure and to collect the material after the curette has been introduced into the endometrial cavity. In one study, the uterine Explora curette was found to have the same diagnostic accuracy as conventional D&C [109].

4.1.1.3. Vacuum Pump (Electric Suction Devices)
Vabra Aspirator

The vacuum curettage was described by Jensen [87] in 1968. This instrument combines vacuum and abrasion, and was accordingly named 'Vabra'. It consists of a stainless steel or rigid plastic cannula with an outside diameter of 3 mm. The suction is started by a device that generates a 600-mm-Hg vacuum.

Results of the Technique

In 1982, Grimes [69] compared D&C with the Vabra aspirator and concluded that 'D&C probably should not be the primary procedure used for obtaining most samples of endometrium'. Because of its smaller diameter than the conventional curette, the Vabra was better tolerated than the D&C, did not require anesthetic, had few complications and could be used in the office. In spite of the fact that the method was easy to learn, economical and reliable, it has not become widely used. One of the disadvantages of Vabra curettage is the need for a vacuum pump and that the high negative pressure can cause discomfort to some women. Techniques using manually applied suction by means of a syringe or a plunger in the cannula have replaced the Vabra technique.

Other Electric Suction Devices

Other devices with a vacuum pump have been described, like the Masterson Endometrial Biopsy System, composed of a stainless steel cannula similar to Novak's curette with a reusable hand-operated pump rather than a syringe, or the Tis-U-Trap, made of flexible plastic with a self-contained tissue filter, and an external suction source. Theses devices are almost out of use [105].

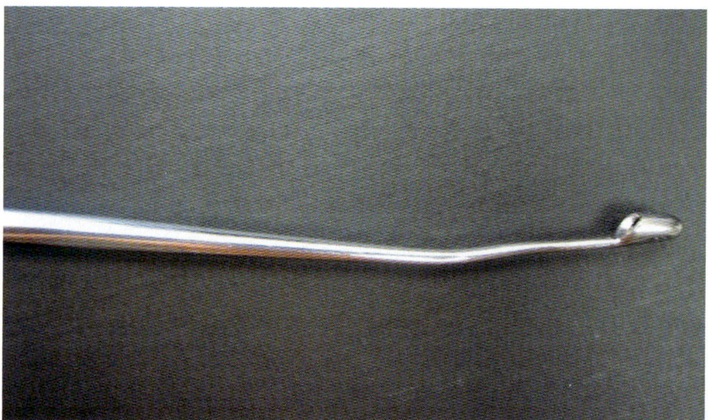

Fig. 4.4. Curette used for D&C.

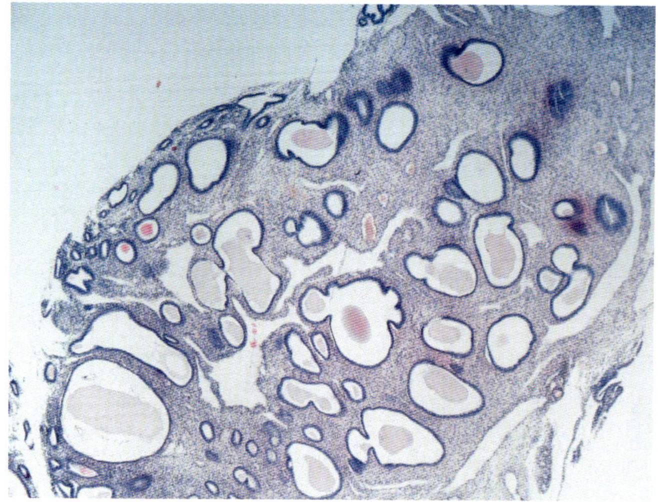

Fig. 4.5. Polyps may be missed during D&C.

Table 4.5. Disadvantages of D&C

– Blind procedure
– Mechanical dilatation often performed
– Requires an operating room which increases the cost of care
– The woman usually receives general anesthesia, increasing both her risk and recovery time

4.1.2. Brushing Technique

Milan and Markley [134] described the Mimark helix in 1973. The material obtained by scraping the inner wall of the uterus is more suitable for cytological than for histological examination.

Results of the Technique

Although the Mimark sampling was well tolerated, the proportion of inadequate samples was reported to be up to 40% for histological specimens and 30% for cytological specimens and the technique has therefore not been widely used [44].

4.2. Dilatation and Curettage

D&C is generally performed under general anesthesia although a local or spinal anesthesia may be an alternative. The procedure is usually done in a hospital or clinic but does not require an overnight stay. After the speculum is inserted in the vagina, the cervix is gradually dilated. A curette (small spoon-shaped instrument) is then guided through the cervix and into the uterus (fig. 4.4). The top layer of the lining of the uterus is carefully scraped off and removed for biopsy (table 4.5).

Results of the Technique

D&C is still considered the gold standard approach in the investigation of patients with abnormal uterine bleeding. This is particularly true for women with post-menopausal bleeding and an endometrium 5 mm or more in thickness since endometrial pathology is present in about 60% of these women [103].

The two main problems associated with D&C are focal lesions of the endometrium and the correct grading of carcinoma.

In one study the agreement between the D&C diagnosis and the final diagnosis was unacceptably poor (59%) in women with focal endometrial pathology detected at hysteroscopy, whereas the agreement was excellent (94%) in women with diffuse involvement [60]. In another study comprising both pre- and postmenopausal women with abnormal uterine bleeding, 40–90% of polyps and 43–66% of hyperplasias were missed by D&C (fig. 4.5) [212]. The grading of carcinoma is another important problem. The hysterectomy histopathologic tumor grade and depth of myometrial invasion both correlate strongly with the prevalence of lymph node metastases and survival in patients with endometrial cancer. Because of the difficulty in accurately predicting depth of myometrial invasion preoperatively, tumor grade has been the main measurable preoperative parameter used to guide surgical management in staging patients with endometrial cancer. Unfortunately, tumor grade based on preoperative endometrial biopsy does not always agree with the grading on the hysterectomy specimen (fig. 4.6). Larson et al. [117] found that D&C incorrectly graded approximately 25% of the patients, with a higher grade tumor being missed in about 10%.

Techniques of Endometrial Histopathology

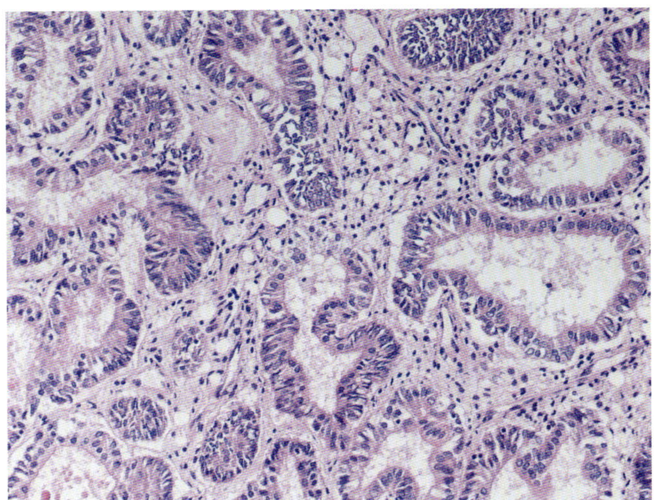

Fig. 4.6. A grade 1 endometrioid carcinoma was diagnosed after D&C. The hysterectomy specimen showed solid areas and a grade 2 adenocarcinoma.

4.3. Hysteroscopy and Curettage

Hysteroscopy uses a hysteroscope, which is a thin telescope connected to a light source to illuminate the area to be visualized, and that is inserted through the cervix into the uterus. Because the inside of the uterus is a potential cavity, it is necessary to distend it with either a liquid (saline, sorbitol, or a dextran solution) or a gas (carbon dioxide) in order to visualize the endometrium. After cervical dilation, the hysteroscope is guided into the uterine cavity and an inspection is performed. If abnormalities are found, an operative hysteroscope also has a channel to allow specialized instruments to enter the cavity and perform surgery. Usually a hysteroscopic intervention is done under anesthesia, but a diagnostic procedure can be performed without anesthesia with instruments of smaller caliber. Rigid hysteroscopes are the

Table 4.6. Advantages of hysteroscopy and curettage

- Macroscopic assessment of the whole uterine cavity and its pathology
- Better results in postmenopausal women (because of atrophic changes of the endometrium)
- Direct biopsy in the detection of early stages of endometrial cancer or endometrial hyperplasia, especially focal lesions

most commonly used instruments. Their wide range of diameters allows for in-office and complex operating-room procedures. The flexible hysteroscope is most commonly used for office hysteroscopy (table 4.6).

Results of the Technique

Nowadays, hysteroscopy-guided biopsy or curettage is probably the most accurate method of assessing the endometrium. Office procedures can be performed easily and inexpensively in an initial evaluation. However, if insufficient material is obtained, if symptoms persist or if focal lesions are suspected, hysteroscopy and curettage should be performed [21].

Endometrial polyps and hyperplasia, although benign, should be correctly diagnosed and removed. Firstly, because the benign pathology may be the cause of the postmenopausal bleeding and if it is not properly removed symptoms may persist, resulting in repeated diagnostic procedures. Secondly, because some studies indicate that both polyps and hyperplasia are risk factors for developing endometrial cancer [168].

Operative hysteroscopy should be considered as an alternative of D&C, especially if focal lesions are present. Some authors consider hysteroscopy the method of choice for the diagnosis of endometrial and endouterine disease, since they believe that blind procedures have no place in the diagnosis of uterine disorders [14].

Chapter 5

New Techniques for the Diagnosis of Endometrial Pathology

Introduction

In developed countries, endometrial cancer (EC) is the commonest neoplasia of the female genital tract, representing almost 50% of all genital cancers. It is becoming increasingly common due to rising living standards, changing eating habits, the aging of the population, hormonal treatments, etc., developing into one of the diseases of modern life [83].

75–80% of cases of cancer of the endometrium occur in postmenopausal women, in particular among women between 60 and 70 years of age, only 3–5% occur in women under 40.

We know that 80–95% of these cancers are first manifested by postmenopausal metrorrhagia. However, postmenopausal metrorrhagia is a frequent cause of gynecological consultation (approx. 5–7.5%) but only 10–15% is due to EC.

While the detection of cervical or breast cancer is based on screening programs applied to the general population or to high-risk populations, EC does not lend itself to the same diagnostic techniques. The general population will not benefit from screening programs, partly as prevalence is not high enough (10–20 cases/100,000 women/year) and partly because its preclinical phase is quite short (4–6.6 years) [107]. However, certain high-risk groups do exist which may benefit from the application of diagnostic techniques when the patients are still at an asymptomatic stage [183] (table 5.1)

For decades fractioned curettage was the preferred method for diagnosing EC, but, apart from being an invasive method, requiring both anesthesia and hospitalization, it was not free of diagnostic error (2–6% false-negatives) in particular for focal lesions such as polyps, focal hyperplasia or minor carcinomas of the endometrium. The appearance of new ambulatory diagnostic methods such as the vaginal ultrasound scan (TS), endometrial aspiration and hysteroscopy have replaced the diagnostic curettage not only in the management of postmenopausal metrorrhagia but also as a screening method for asymptomatic women, since these methods are all simpler, cheaper and less invasive.

Diagnostic Methods for Endometrial Pathology

5.1. Ultrasound

Abdominal ultrasound scans allow an overall evaluation of the uterus and its relation to the various pelvic organs, but it is not a method of screening for endometrial pathology.

Although TS was initially limited to sterility, it is currently used in day-to-day gynecological practice. The transvaginal probe has a higher resolution as it moves closer to the internal genital apparatus. It is a simple, and economical method (offering excellent value for money), which is also reliable, risk-free and easy on the patient. It provides information not only concerning the endometrium, but also on the

Table 5.1. SEGO – Carcinoma of the Endometrium: Consensus Conference on Prevention of Female Cancer (Coordinator: Prof. R. Comino Delgado), Cadiz 1997

	Score 0	Score 1	Score 2
Age, years	<50	50–60	>65
Nulliparity	No	No	Yes
Obesity	IMC <25	IMC = 25–27	IMC >27
Diabetes mellitus	No	No	Yes
Estrogen therapy not compensated for by progesterone	No	No	Yes
Tamoxifen	No	<2 years	>2 years

Low risk = 0 points, medium risk = 1–2 points, high risk >3 points.

New Techniques for the Diagnosis of Endometrial Pathology

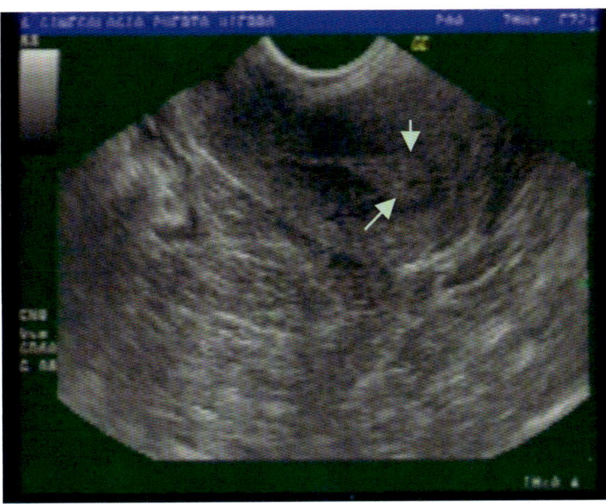

Fig. 5.1. Longitudinal cut of the uterus to measure the ETh.

myometrium and the ovaries. Being an immediately available diagnostic resource (in many centers it is kept in the gynecological examinations room) it is presently the primary and most important screening tool in the early diagnosis of endometrial pathology in women with postmenopausal metrorrhagia.

Two aspects are considered in the transvaginal ultrasound examination of the endometrium: *endometrial thickness* and *endometrial morphology or sonostructure*.

Endometrial Thickness (ETh)

This is based on the fact that EC is almost always associated with a thick and irregular endometrium and is rarely seen in a thin endometrium. TS scans allow us to study the whole endometrial cavity and to select those cases that require a histological study.

We are dealing with a quantitative, objective variable and measurements are reproducible from one radiologist to another. Measurement of ETh is not difficult when certain norms are observed; a longitudinal cut is made of the uterus and the endometrium is measured at the point of maximum thickness, including the two endometrial layers and excluding the subendometrial hyposonogenic line that corresponds to the innermost layer of the myometrium (fig. 5.1).

However, there are several factors that can influence the evaluation of ETh: the phase of the menstrual cycle, obesity, hypertension, menopausal years, symptoms, hormonal treatment, etc.

In premenopausal women, parallel to the hormonal changes accompanying the menstrual cycle, endometrial changes occur that are reflected in the ultrasound image. Thus, the endometrium in the follicular phase appears as a thin ultrasonogenic layer, which grows by approximately 0.5 mm/day reaching 9–14 mm in the secretory phase.

In postmenopausal women, the level of ETh that should be considered as pathological varies with the presence or absence of symptoms and with the number of years since menopause. It is necessary to determine a level of ETh below which there is no real probability of endometrial malignancy in women with postmenopausal bleeding. In Smith-Bindman's [195] classic meta-analysis of 85 studies published between 1966 and 1996, which included a total of 5,892 women with ETh >5 mm, the sensitivity was 96% and the specificity 68% for the diagnosis of endometrial pathology. The risk of EC in a woman with postmenopausal metrorrhagia and an ETh of <5 mm, measured by TS, is less than 1% according to several authors. It would thus appear to be reasonable not to perform more invasive investigations in these cases. On the other hand, histological examination is indicated in cases in which the endometrium is >5 mm thick. Furthermore, the positive predictive value of the TS increases with the ETh. Karlsson et al. [103] found the prevalence of EC to be 2.2% when ETh was 5 mm, 19.3% when thickness was ≥8 mm and 57.1% when it was ≥20 mm.

The incidence of hidden or asymptomatic EC is low – between 1.3 and 1.7 per 1,000 postmenopausal women. In some countries the use of ETh measured by TS as a screening technique used in asymptomatic postmenopausal women has been rejected due to cost considerations, that is to say, in the light of cost/benefit. However, the increasing frequency of this type of cancer and of the proportion of postmenopausal adults increases the need for an early diagnosis. More and more studies demonstrate the utility of TS scan as a routine diagnostic method, but not with the cut value of Eth used in the asymptomatic postmenopausal women.

Endometrial Sonostructure

Various endometrial sonomorphologies correspond more or less well with different endometrial pathologies. The specificity and the positive predictive value of the TS can be improved by adding an assessment of endometrial texture.

Endometrial polyps (EP) are described ultrasonically as one or more intraluminal formations, which may vary in size, are rounded, hypersonogenic, homogeneous and well-defined, and which on occasions are separated from the surrounding endometrium by a sononegative halo.

Endometrial hyperplasia (EH) presents as a diffuse endometrial thickening of variable sonogenicity (homogeneous, hypo- or ultrasonogenic or irregular).

A myoma is seen as a nodular, ultrasonogenic formation with a non-homogeneous texture, which usually leaves a posterior shadow. The TS allows us to determine both the number and size of myomas, to evaluate the intramural extension of the submucosal myomas and to measure the surgical

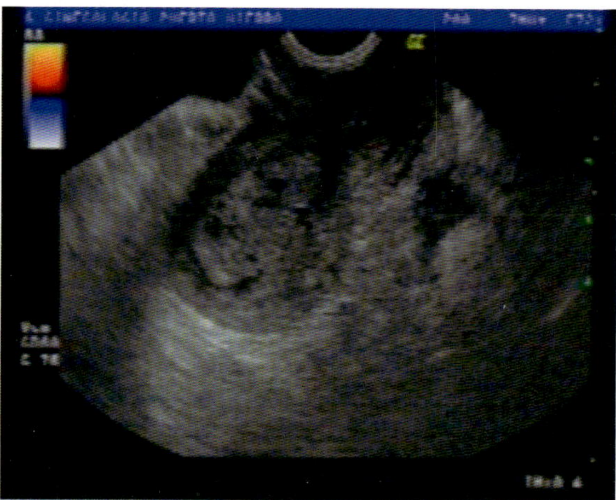

Fig. 5.2. Suspicious pattern: uterine cavity occupied by a non-homogeneous endometrium with irregular borders.

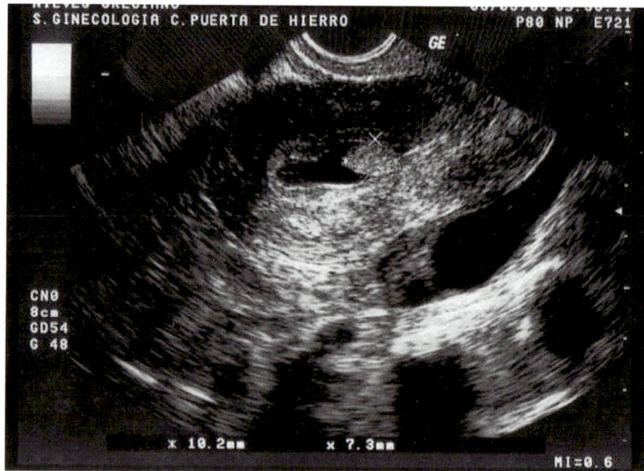

Fig. 5.3. Sagittal cut of the uterus where a cavity, distended by saline serum, can be seen around an endometrial polyp.

safety margin, that is, the distance between the external surface of a myoma and the uterine serosa (this being crucial to the evaluation of the possibility of hysteroscopic resection).

Although there are no specific patterns for each type of endometrial pathology, we should mention a non-homogeneous endometrium that is ultrasonogenic, has an irregular border to the myometrium, irregular liquid areas, and an ultrasonogenic halo, among the sonomorphologic parameters suspected of malignancy (fig. 5.2).

However, assessment of endometrial sonostructure, apart from being subjective and difficult to measure, depends on the experience of the ultrasound technician and on the characteristics of the scan, and is more time-consuming.

5.2. Hysterosonography

This is a painless invasive technique causing little patient discomfort that allows the complete visualization of the uterine cavity, which has been distended by the previous introduction of saline serum through a catheter placed in the endocervical canal (fig. 5.3). This is a test in real time that complements the TS when this has not been conclusive. It increases the predictive value of the ultrasound scan in the diagnosis of intracavital pathology [59].

5.3. Color Doppler and Pulsed Doppler

This permits the study in real time of the sanguineous flow through the endometrium, enhancing both the predictive and diagnostic ability of the ultrasound scan.

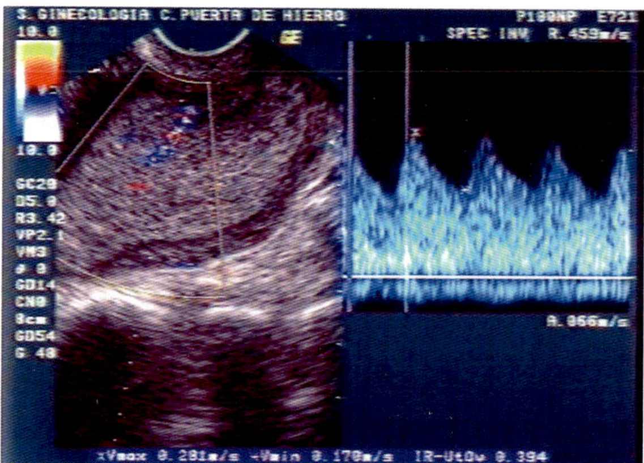

Fig. 5.4. Presence of vascularization in an endometrium suspected to be malignant. A Doppler of newly formed endometrial vessels. Very high diastolic flows and very low RI (0.39) are noted.

The color Doppler (fig. 5.4) can identify the presence of tumoral neoangiogenesis (necessary for the tumor to grow) while the pulsed Doppler shows us the characteristics of the speed wave from the flow of these vascular signals, which, being newly formed, have low peripheral resistance and high diastolic blood flow. These parameters are measured as indexes of resistance (RI) and pulse (PI).

We can thus visualize and measure the RI of the uterine, arcuate, radial and spiral arteries. We can also look for the vascular pedicle that supplies an EP, or demonstrate the peripheral vascular distribution of submucosal myomas. The presence of intratumoral and myometrial endometrial vessels with low vascular resistance suggests malignancy [58].

New Techniques for the Diagnosis of
Endometrial Pathology

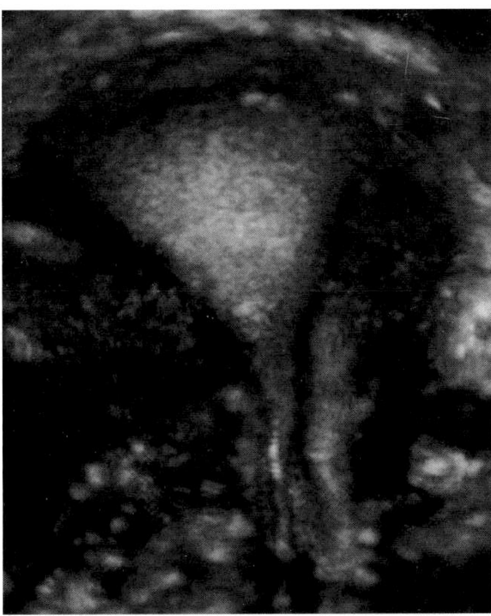

Fig. 5.5. Coronal cut of the uterus, showing simultaneously the endometrium of the uterine horns and the cervix.

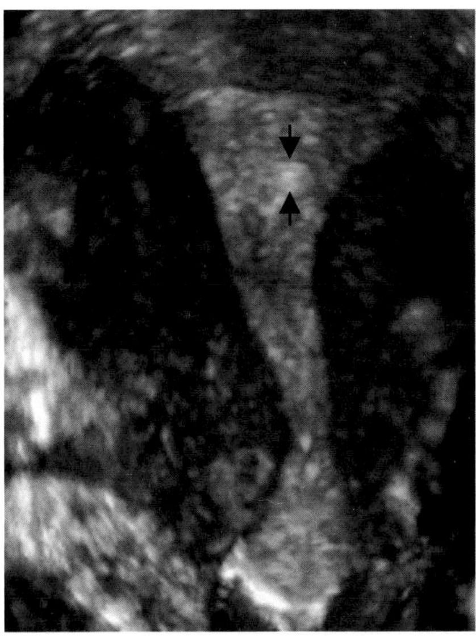

Fig. 5.6. Focal thickening of an endometrium: as well as evaluating its volume and position, we can see the existence or not of myometrial invasion.

Power Doppler or 'color Doppler energy' have recently been introduced in clinical practice. These are more sensitive to lower speed flows and give us a clearer picture of the vascular architecture.

5.4. 3D Ultrasound (fig. 5.5, 5.6)

These are ultrasound scans that use higher speed sound waves to create an image and that allow for the later treatment of the image. We can now use what are called 4D, which give a three-dimensional image almost in real time.

The three-dimensional ultrasound scan not only lets us study ETh, but also the volume of the endometrium and the extension and level of invasion of tumors [110].

5.5. Hysteroscopy in the Office

This is, at the present time, the 'gold standard' in the diagnosis of endometrial pathology as it allows the direct observation of the endometrium and the taking of directed biopsies [132]. It is a simple invasive technique, easily learnt, quick and effective, highly dependent on the clinician and with some complications or risks that can be minimized by training and experience.

It not only allows us to take directed biopsies but to treat certain lesions directly, all this in the clinic and with minimal discomfort to the patient. A rigid stainless steel telescope is used, which is 25 cm long and 4 mm thick and has a 30° lens at one end and a cold light column and viewing lens at the other end (fig. 5.7). Adequate hysteroscopic examination requires distension of the uterine cavity. This is achieved by one of two methods: gaseous or liquid distension. Saline serum is generally used as it is readily available, cheap, easily absorbed by the peritoneum, of low toxicity and gives good endoscopic vision.

The hysteroscope has a complementary channel that permits the use of several instruments such as scissors, tweezers or electrodes, which let us perform minor operations such as the removal of EP, the use of intrauterine devices, the sectioning of adhesions, or directed biopsies.

A great variety of endometrial images are seen in premenopausal women, which are not visible after the menopause. For this reason, hysteroscopy is far easier in postmenopausal women in whom atrophy is the commonest pattern, than in premenopausal patients.

The *atrophic* endometrium looks like a smooth, thin, transparent epithelium which lets us see the underlying vascular structures and is easy to study. In postmenopausal women, any endometrium that has not atrophied must be biopsied (fig. 5.8).

An EP is seen as an exophytic lesion, which is soft with a smooth surface and poor vascularization. It is important to observe all the faces of the EP as well as the surrounding endometrium. The number, size, position and base of any polyps can be assessed (fig. 5.9).

Myomas are lumps of different sizes with a pearly surface and a hard consistency. Vessels of varying calibers are seen

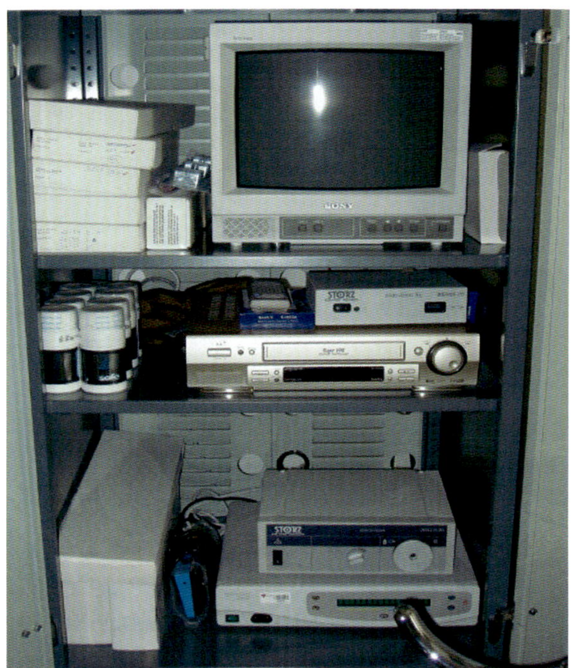

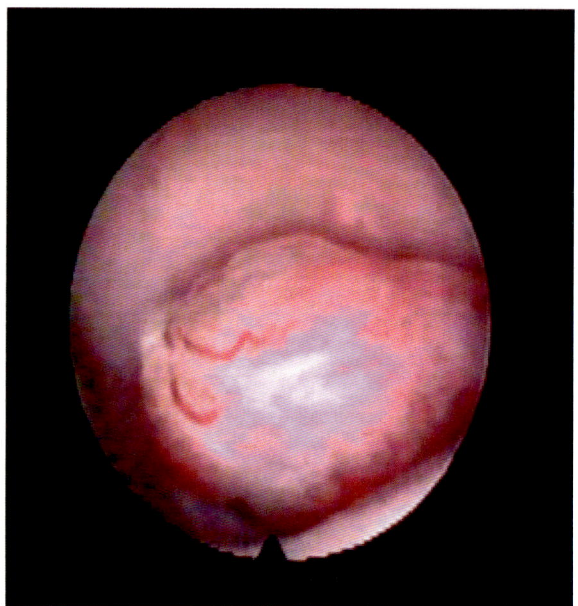

Fig. 5.9. Cavity occupied by an endometrial polyp.

Fig. 5.7. Hysteroscopic column in the office: the cupboard has shelves to hold the following elements, from the top down: monitor, video camera, video recorder, a light source and the irrigation pump.

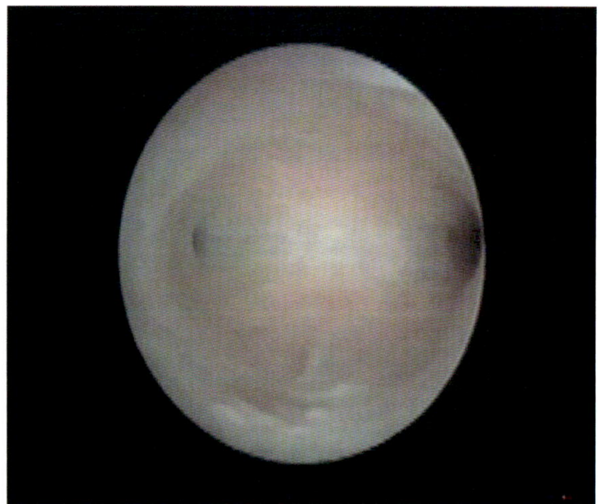

Fig. 5.8. Uterine cavity with atrophic endometrium.

on the surface. It is possible to decide the number, size, position and especially the proportion of intracavital extension of myomas (evaluating the angle formed between the edge of the myoma and the uterine cavity). The European Society of Hysteroscopy uses the Wamsteker and De Block classification, which subdivides myomas on the basis of the percentage of intramural extension: type 0: the myoma is pedunculated or sessile, 100% submucosal; type I: over 50% of the myoma is submucosal, and type II: less than 50% is submucosal (not accessible to hysteroscopic surgery).

EH is a histologically defined lesion that may have no hysteroscopic equivalent. This explains the low sensitivity of hysteroscopy in the diagnosis of EH. We may see a greatly thickened endometrium with a wavy or polypoid surface, a high glandular density and increased vascularization.

Compression with the hysteroscope may leave a deep mark. Unfortunately we have not been able to define a hysteroscopic image that corresponds to all the histological characteristics of the EH. For this reason, in practical clinical hysteroscopy, EH is simply divided into low- and high-risk EH (assessing the risk of malignant changes).

In EC, the hysteroscope allows confirmation of the diagnosis with almost 100% accuracy, and a specificity of 95%. Macroscopically, it may appear to be diffuse or focal depending on whether more or less than 50% of the cavity is affected. In hysteroscopic terms, two types of EC can be distinguished. In the hormone-dependent type, the endometrium appears thickened and polypoid with atypical hypervascularization and areas of necrosis. In the non-hormone-dependent type there is a compact tumor resembling an EP or a hypervascularized myoma, which is surrounded by an atrophic endometrium (fig. 5.10).

New Techniques for the Diagnosis of
Endometrial Pathology

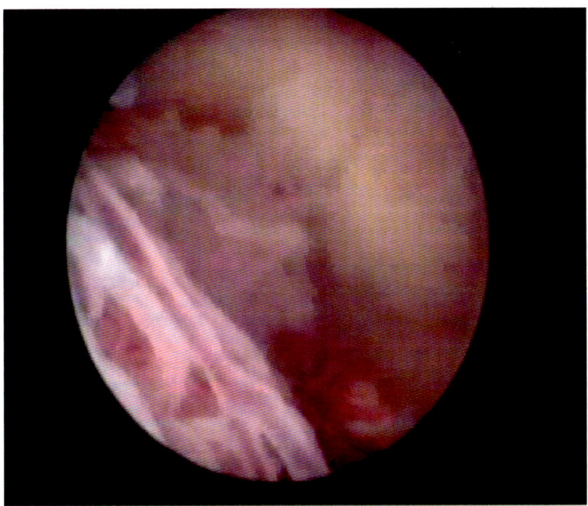

Fig. 5.10. Cancer of the endometrium: endometrium with atypical vascularization.

However, hysteroscopy is not an accurate method for pre-operative evaluation of the depth of myometrial invasion and of cervical stroma invasion.

In summary, the range of tests we have described are indeed useful tools in the diagnosis of endometrial pathology. The uterine cavity, inaccessible as it is to the human eye, presents diagnostic difficulties that are partly resolved by the use of the techniques considered here. These techniques allow us to confirm or suggest a diagnosis, which is usually confirmed by histological study of the endometrium. These tests carry no risks and can be performed in outpatients with a sensitivity and a specificity that varies according to the type of endometrial pathology present. They are complementary to existing methods and have a clinical value that should not be underestimated.

Chapter 6

Cytology of the Normal Endometrium – Cycling and Postmenopausal

6.1. Histology of the Endometrium

The uterine corpus is composed of a modified mucosa known as the endometrium, a fibromuscular wall called the myometrium, and a serosal lining. The uterine mucosa can be divided into two regions: the mucosa of the lower uterine segment (LUS) (isthmus) and the mucosa of the corpus proper (fig. 6.1). The mucosa of the LUS, located between the endocervix and endometrium, is thinner than that of the fundus and its glands respond only slightly to hormonal stimulation. There is a gradual morphologic transition from the isthmic mucosa to the endocervical mucosa.

During the reproductive years the endometrium of the corpus proper undergoes regular cyclic changes as a response to the release of the ovarian hormones, estrogen and progesterone.

The endometrium consists of simple tubular glands set in a cellular vascular stroma. It is composed of a thin basal layer (basalis), which abuts on the myometrium, and a functional layer on top of the basalis. The functional layer is highly responsive to hormonal ovarian influence in contrast to the basalis. The functional endometrium consists of a superficial layer with few glands and abundant stroma (the compacta), and a deep layer that has many glands and relatively less stroma (the spongiosa) (fig. 6.2).

The structure and activity of a functional endometrium reflect the pattern of ovarian hormone secretion. The histologic types of glandular cells are columnar or cuboid. The endometrium undergoes regular growth and maturation and when the cycle ends, in the absence of pregnancy, shedding occurs followed by regeneration. The average duration of the cycle is 28 days. In a normal cycle the postovulatory phase lasts 14 days. Changes in the length of the cycle are usually due to the duration of the proliferative phase, which can vary from 8 to 21 days [47].

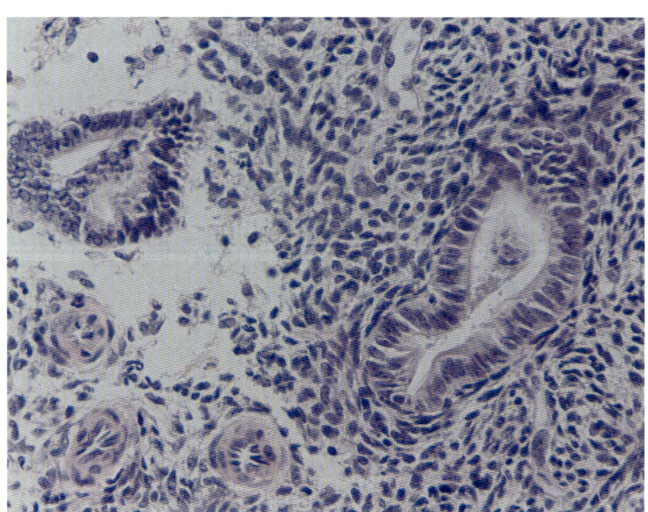

Fig. 6.1. Histology of endometrium. Cell block: HE, 40×.

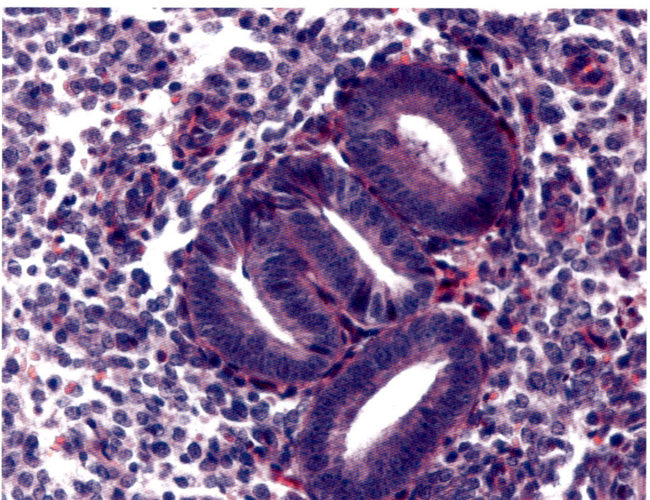

Fig. 6.2. Functional layer of endometrium glands and stroma. Cell block: HE, 40×.

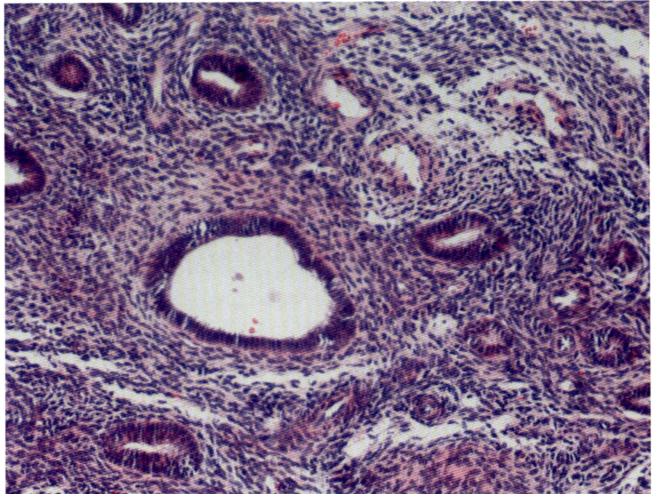

Fig. 6.3. Stroma of the endometrium. Histology: HE, 20×.

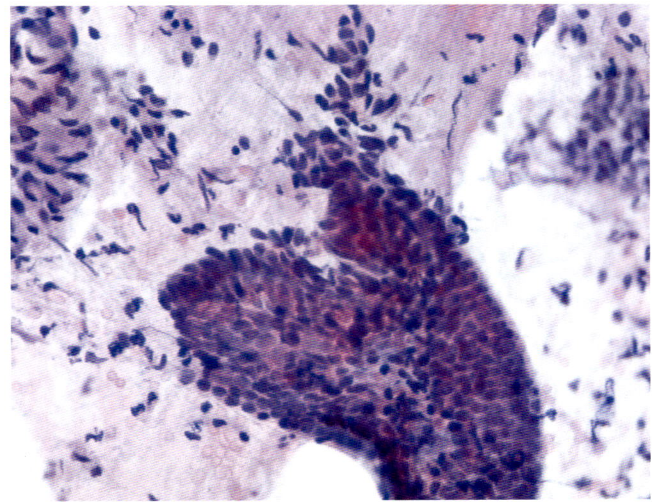

Fig. 6.4. Components of endometrial smear. Pap, 20×.

The Glands of the Endometrium. The endometrial glands are simple tubular glands lined by columnar epithelium or tall, narrow and closely packed cells with elongated and parallel nuclei (fig. 6.2). The morphology of the endometrial glands changes during the different phases of the menstrual cycle.

The Stroma of the Endometrium. The endometrial stroma consists of pluripotential mesenchymal cells, which at the beginning of the menstrual cycle are spindle-shaped, poorly differentiated and joined to one another by cytoplasmic processes (fig. 6.3). The cells lie firmly anchored within a network of reticulum fibers. At the beginning of the cycle the cytoplasm of the cells forms a narrow ring around the nuclei. Towards the end of the proliferative phase the nuclear chromatine becomes less dense. During the secretory phase vacuoles and granulocytes appear in the cytoplasm, and some of the cells differentiate into predecidual cells.

The stroma of the basalis is more cellular than that of the functional layer of the endometrium and nucleocytoplasmic ratios are high. Thick-walled arteries, lymphocytes and lymphoid aggregates are present.

6.2. The Endometrial Smear

A smear obtained by endometrial brushing techniques (EBT) of the normal endometrium is composed of large sheets of surface epithelial cells in a honeycomb pattern with gland openings, and poorly cohesive stromal cells with oval nuclei and ill-defined cytoplasm. There are histiocytes, granulocytes and red blood cells mixed with cell fragments and mucus in the smear background. Tumoral diathesis is absent (fig. 6.4).

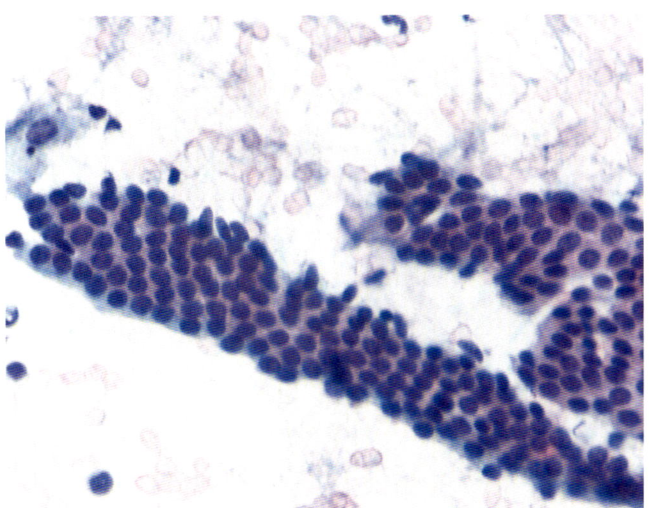

Fig. 6.5. Endometrial epithelial cells. Pap, 40×.

Endometrial Epithelial Cells

The cells of endometrial glands and surface epithelium present the same morphology, both are columnar or cylindrical. Their morphology changes from the proliferative to the secretory phase. Ciliated glandular cells can be identified in a few cases, often in estrogen-stimulated endometrium.

Endometrial epithelial cells occur in sheets or cohesive groups, seldom with a honeycomb pattern. Isolated cells are common. They show little variation in size and shape with scant cytoplasm and round, ovoid or elongated nuclei with dense chromatin. Nucleoli are usually not visible. Cell borders are ill-defined (fig. 6.5). Mitotic figures are common in the proliferative phase. The morphology seen in the secretory phased is described below.

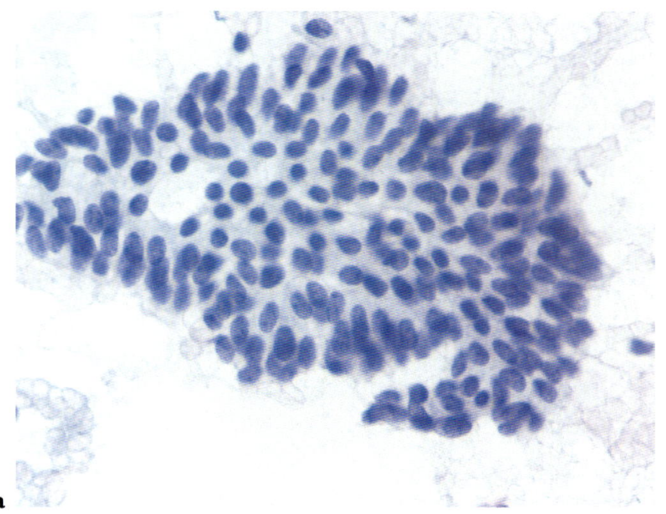 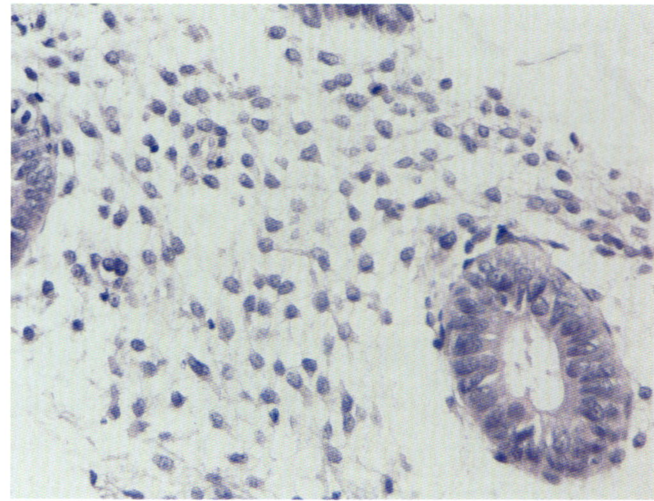

a

b

Fig. 6.6. LBP of endometrium. **a** Cytology: Pap, 40×, and **b** cell block: HE, 40×.

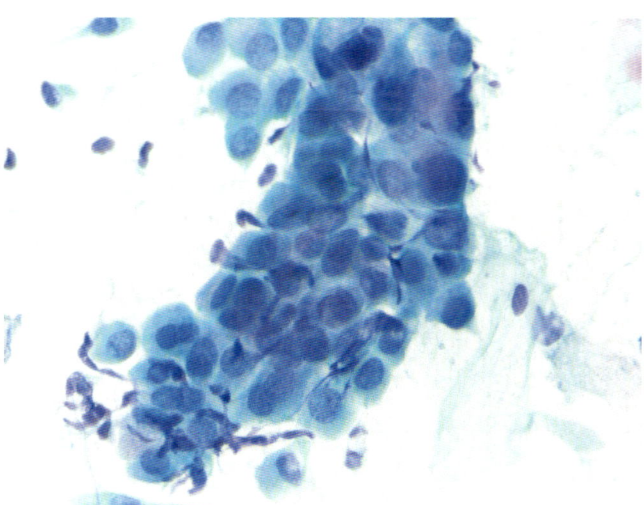 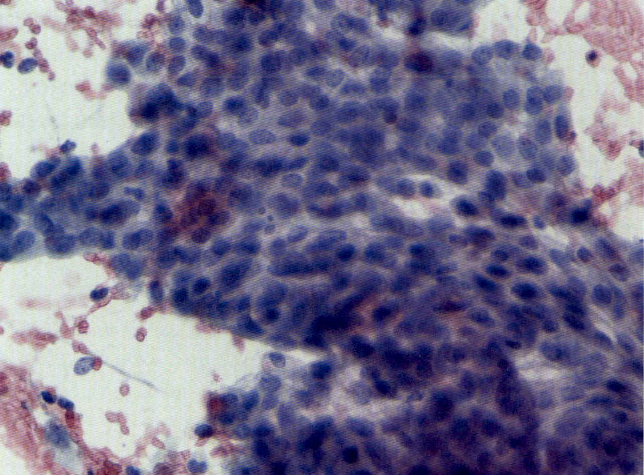

Fig. 6.7. Smear of LUS. Pap, 60×.

Fig. 6.8. Stromal cells of the endometrium. Proliferative phase. Endometrial brushing: Pap, 40×.

In liquid-based samples (LBP) endometrial cells may appear more hyperchromatic and more pleomorphic with somewhat more prominent nucleoli than in conventional smears (fig. 6.6). In general, the improved diagnostic yield of LBP tests may be attributed to better cell preservation and the absence of obscuring blood or inflammation that is often encountered in conventional smears. This allows the detection of even low numbers of diagnostic cells on LBP tests.

The glandular cells derived from direct sampling of the LUS include larger groups with gland openings, branched glands and nuclear palisading within the fragments accompanied by endometrial stroma [76] (fig. 6.7).

Stromal Cells of the Endometrium

The endometrial stromal cells are mesodermal cells, mainly of fibroblastic, seldom of histiocytic type. In the endometrial brush smears the morphology of the endometrial stromal cells varies with the clinical status of the patient and with the phase of the menstrual cycle. In the early proliferative phase the stromal cells occur singly or in loose groupings, they have scant cytoplasm and ovoid or fusiform nuclei (fig. 6.8). In the late proliferative and early secretory phases the stromal cells appear as more cohesive groups of spindle cells (fig. 6.9). Variable degrees of predecidualization, form small isolated stromal cells to large predecidual cells with abundant cytoplasm and ovoid or vesicular nuclei and seldom with obvious nucleoli, can be seen during the later secretory phase.

Cytology of the Normal Endometrium –
Cycling and Postmenopausal

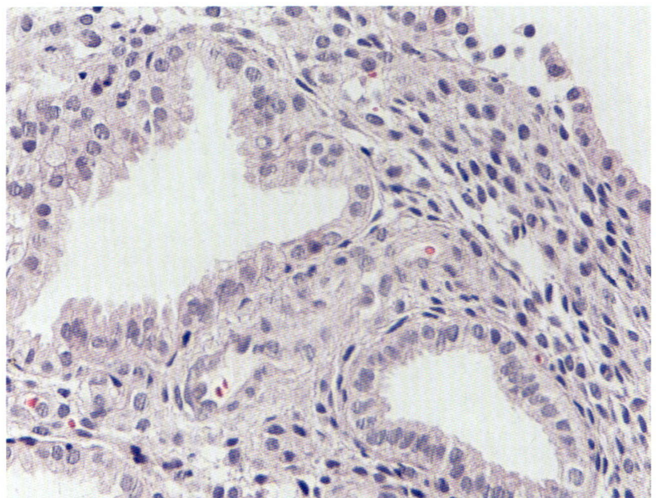

Fig. 6.9. Stromal cells of the endometrium. Secretory phase. Cell block: HE, 40×.

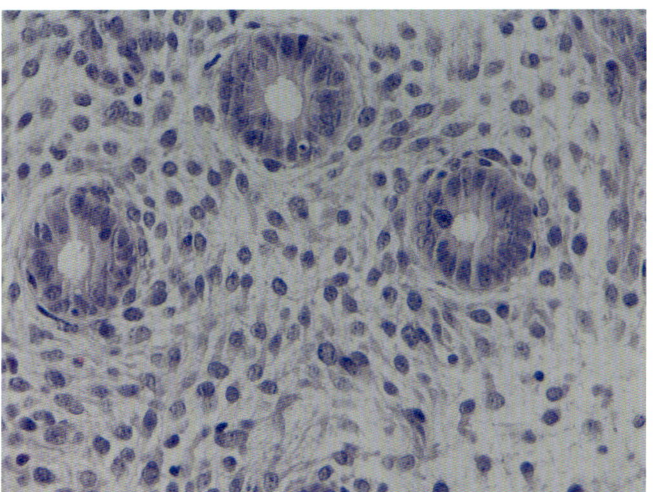

Fig. 6.10. Proliferative phase. Cell block: HE, 40×.

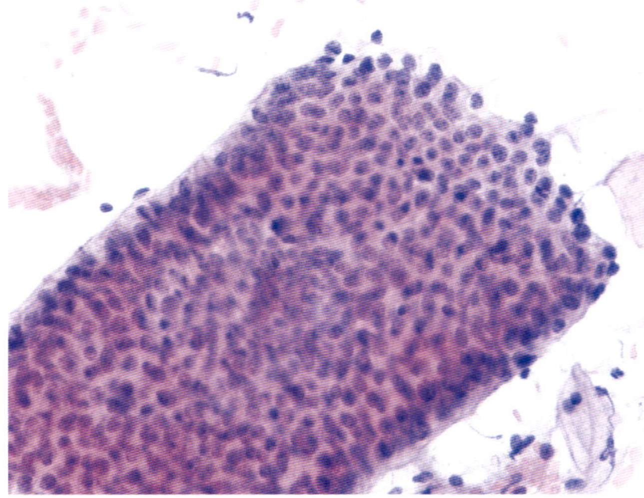

Fig. 6.11. Proliferative phase. Pap, 40×.

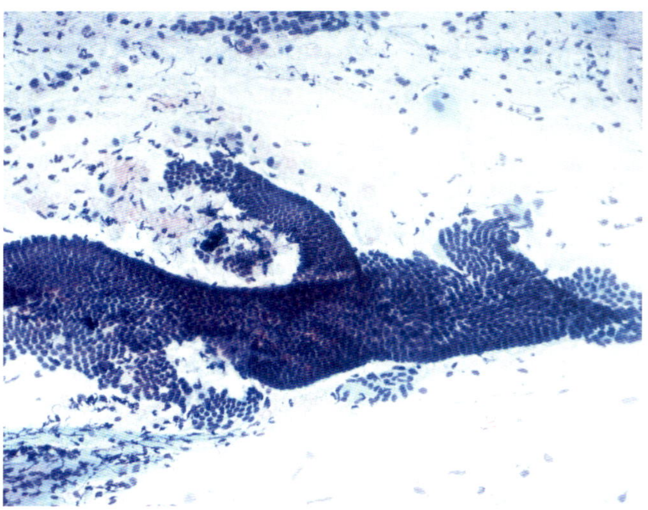

Fig. 6.12. Glove finger in proliferative phase. Pap, 10×.

6.3. Patterns of Normal Endometrial Smears

6.3.1. Endometrial Smear during the Menstrual Cycle

Proliferative Phase

Histology. Estrogenic stimulation causes the endometrium to regenerate and proliferate. In the early proliferative phase the glands are straight and narrow and the glandular epithelium is cubo-columnar. Nuclear chromatin appears dispersed and mitotic figures are present. The stromal cells also show mitotic activity and have ill-defined borders (fig. 6.10). In the late proliferative phase the glands increase in size and appear tortuous with pseudostratification of the epithelium showing nuclei at different levels. The stromal cells are small and spindle-shaped similar to predecidual cells.

Cytology. In the early proliferative phase, EBT show glandular cells in cohesive monolayered sheets. They sometimes appear as straight or twisted tubular structures resembling glove fingers irregularly sheared at the ends, the so-called glove-finger pattern (fig. 6.11) [40]. Almost all the tubular fragments are open at both ends (open type), but a few are closed at one end (closed type) and have a cup-like, a half moon, or spherical shape [160]. The nuclei are of uniform size and shape and have granular chromatin and distinct micronucleoli. Loose aggregates of stromal cells, which have oval nuclei and poorly defined cytoplasm, can be identified. In the late proliferative phase, sheets of endometrial cells are highly cellular with nuclear crowding, denser nuclear chromatin and frequent mitotic figures. Tubular structures are small and a glove-finger pattern is frequently seen (fig. 6.12).

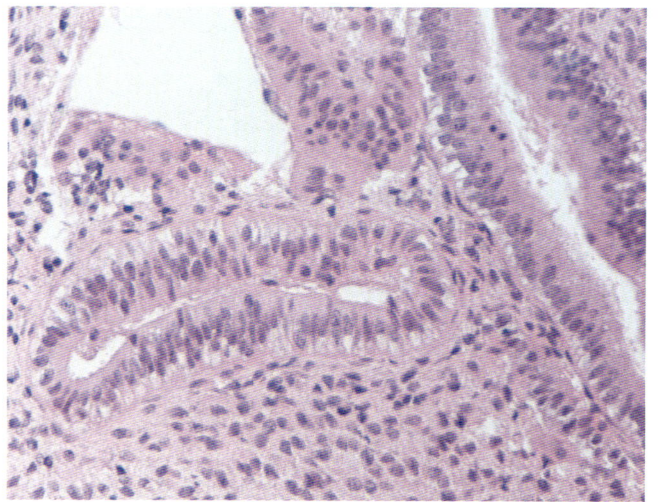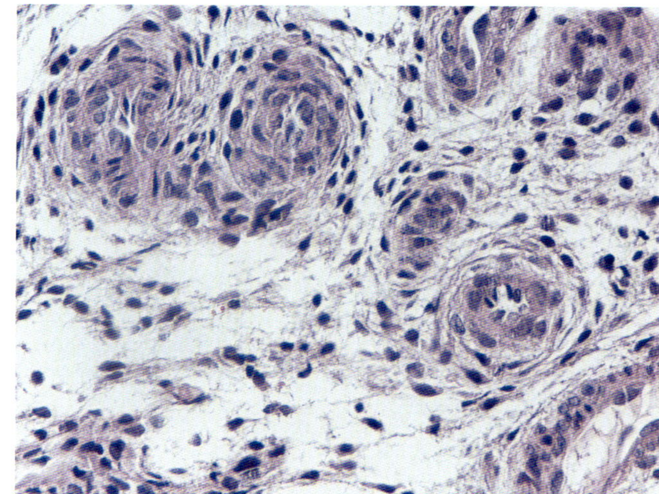

Fig. 6.13. Secretory phase. Histology: **a** subnuclear glycogen vacuoles, HE, 20× and **b** spiral arteries.

Secretory Phase

Histology. During the early secretory phase the endometrium shows the effects of both progesterone and estrogen influence. The endometrial glands undergo progressive distension, appear plumper and more tortuous and are lined by low columnar cells. Subnuclear cytoplasmic glycogen vacuoles may discharge into the gland lumina. In the late secretory phase, stromal cells increase in size and volume and they acquire an epitheloid appearance called predecidual cells. The finding of spiral arteries surrounded by a cuff of predecidual stromal cells is useful in diagnosis (fig. 6.13).

Cytology. In the early secretory phase, the glandular cells become larger with a well-defined clear cytoplasm and a honeycomb pattern. The spindled stromal cells occur in loose or cohesive aggregates. The secretory glandular cells and the stromal predecidual changes are more evident in the late secretory phase (fig. 6.14). The predecidual cells are arranged in small irregular sheets and have abundant dense cytoplasm without vacuolization. Their nuclei have an irregular chromatin structure and visible micronucleoli.

Menstrual Phase

Histology. In the menstrual phase, a plane of separation appears between the superficial endometrium and the basal layer. A variable amount of functional endometrium remains attached to the basalis.

Cytology. EBT produces a bloody smear with many ball-like tissue fragments (menstrual cell balls) consisting of degenerate glandular cells surrounded by predecidual cells [205]. The stromal cells have ovoid, small, pyknotic nuclei and may appear as aggregates. Isolated predecidual cells, neutrophils and nuclear debris are present in the background.

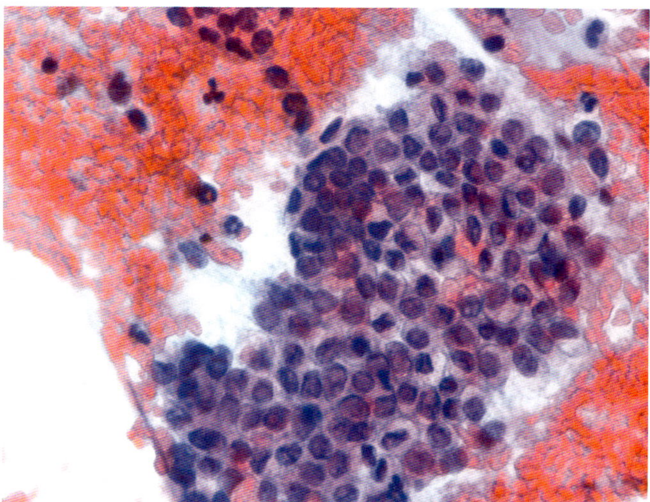

Fig. 6.14. Secretory phase. Pap, 40×.

Cervicovaginal smears have a bloodier and dirtier background with typical exodus, menstrual cell balls and dispersed epithelial and stromal cells (fig. 6.15).

Summary of Endometrial Cytology during the Menstrual Cycle. Based on a review of current knowledge and on more than 35 years' experience using adequate diagnostic criteria, a cytological diagnosis of normal cyclic endometrium is possible with acceptable accuracy (Coscia 92%) [40]. True endometrial dating is more difficult, in our experience impossible. Of greater practical importance is the identification of an early secretory phase in EBT to confirm ovulation. Endometrial cytology has specific problems. A proper cytological training and a good knowledge of the endometrial histopathology in various clinical conditions is necessary to achieve acceptable accuracy.

Cytology of the Normal Endometrium – Cycling and Postmenopausal

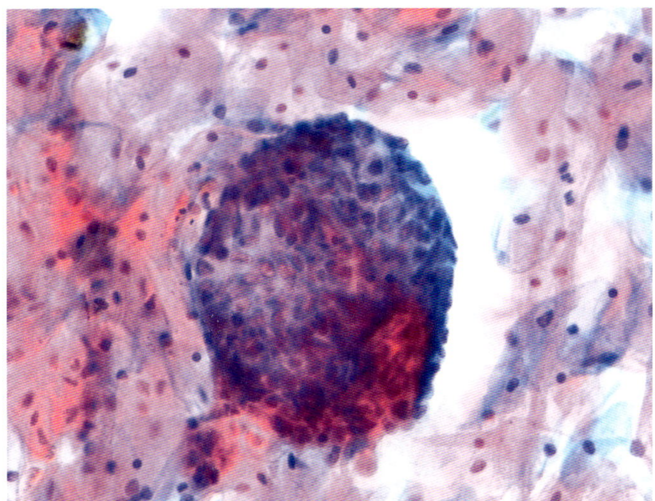

Fig. 6.15. Menstrual phase. Cytology: 'exodus', Pap, 40×.

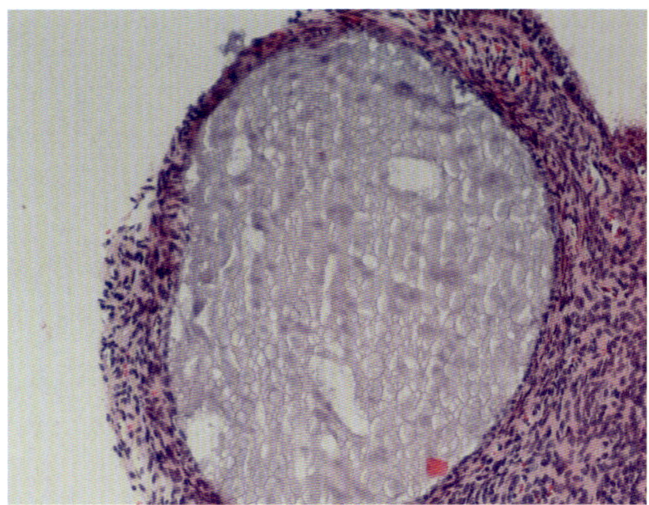

Fig. 6.17. Senile cystic atrophic endometrium. Histology: HE, 20×.

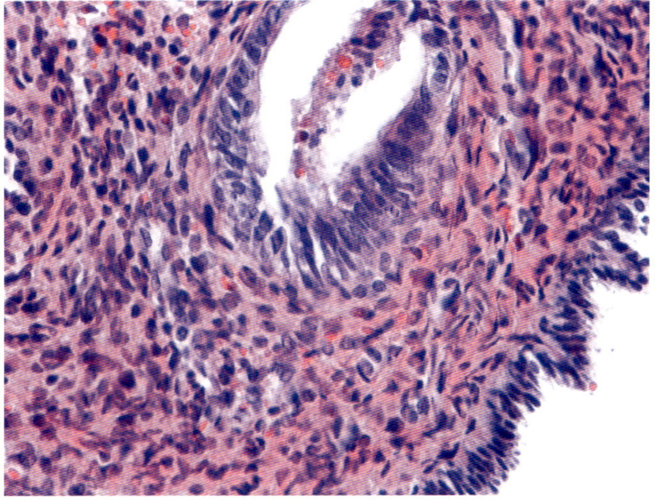

Fig. 6.16. Atrophic endometrium in postmenopausal woman. Histology: HE, 40×.

6.3.2. Endometrial Cytology in the Menopause

Histology. Following the physiological decline of ovarian function with a fall in the secretion of both progesterone and estrogen, the postmenopausal non-functional endometrium usually changes progressively over a few years into an atrophic endometrium (fig. 6.16). But in 20–30% of women this transformation may take several years. We found signs of proliferative endometrial activity in such cases sometimes persisting for many years. It is very important to bear this in mind before prescribing hormone replacement therapy.

Atrophic Endometrium. Since the endometrium is thin, endometrial biopsy samples are often scanty if not inadequate. In more adequate samples there are sparse remnants of narrow glands lined by a low epithelium with small inactive nuclei, supported by a dense fibrous stroma of spindle cells. The functional layer is difficult or impossible to separate from the basalis. More commonly than atrophy, we find signs of weak proliferative activity of the endometrium. In such women, the menopause seems to develop gradually over a few or many years. A third common pattern of menopausal endometrium is seen when the last cycles were anovulatory or had irregular proliferative phases, which results in a senile cystic atrophy (fig. 6.17). The stroma becomes fibrous and the glands vary in size, some of them are narrow and tubular, but many are dilated and cystic. The glandular epithelium is cuboidal and inactive but has a tendency to become polygonal. This histological pattern may be mistaken for glandular-cystic hyperplasia.

Cytology. EBT from *atrophic endometrium* are sparsely cellular containing straight tubular glands and few surface epithelial cells. The epithelial cells are smaller and their appearance is less characteristic and they have a low columnar or cuboidal shape. There are scattered, shrunk stromal cells with scanty cytoplasm. Mitotic figures are absent (fig. 6.18).

In *the weakly proliferative endometrium*, EBT contain glandular cells analogous to those seen in the early proliferative phase of the menstrual cycle, except that there are fewer mitotic figures and the nuclei seem less crowded (fig. 6.19). The *disordered proliferative endometrium of postmenopausal women* usually yields endometrial smears similar to those from the endometrium of the proliferative phase in the reproductive years [205]. In *senile cystic atrophy* EBT produces a moderately cellular smear with few tubular glands and proliferative surface endometrial cells. Scattered stromal cells complete the pattern and distinguish it from cystic hyperplasia.

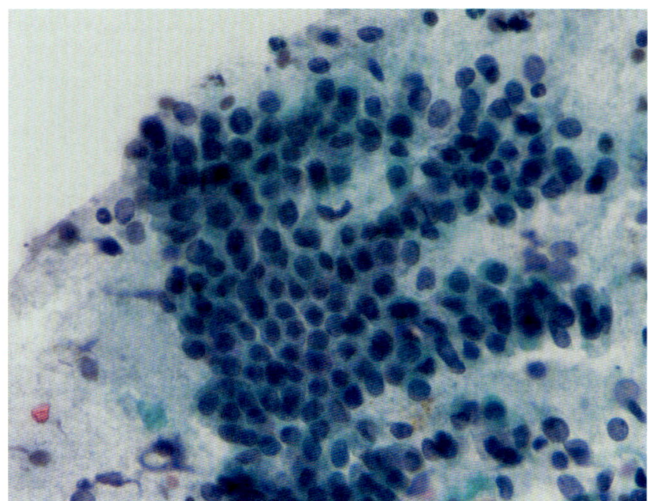

Fig. 6.18. Atrophic endometrium. Pap, 60×.

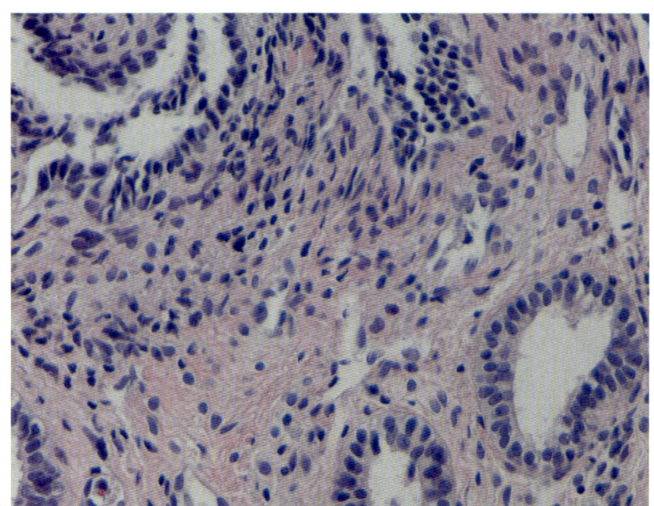

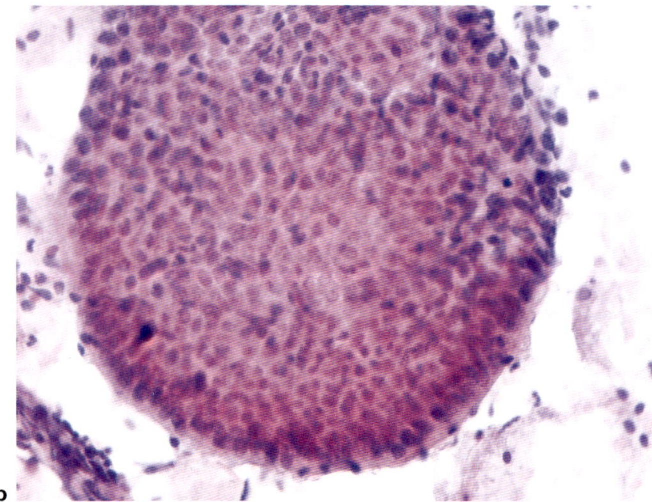

Fig. 6.19. Weakly proliferative endometrium. **a** Cell block: HE, 20× and **b** endometrial brushing: Pap, 20×.

Table 6.1. Differential diagnosis of normal endometrial cells

	Epithelial cells	Stromal cells
Shedding	Large sheets	Loose grouping. Single
Cell pattern	Honeycomb. Tube	Irregular sheets
Type of cell	Columnar. Cylindrical	Fibroblast. Histiocyte
Shape	Round. Oval	Spindle
Nuclei	Round	Oval. Fusiform
Cytoplasm	Dense. Relatively scanty	Ill defined. Predecidual

Table 6.2. Differential diagnosis of endometrial and endocervical cells and histiocytes

	Endometrial	Endocervical	Histiocyte
Cell pattern	Dense sheets	Honeycomb. Palisading	Dispersed
Size	Double that of granulocyte	Larger than endometrial	Great variation
Nuclei	Vary in shape not in size	No variation of shape and size	Variation in shape and size
Cytoplasm	Ill-defined	Well-preserved	Microvacuolization

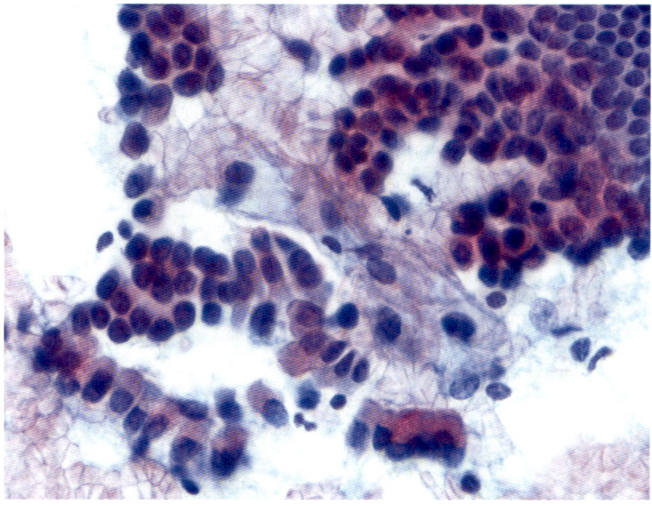

Fig. 6.20. Differential diagnosis with endocervical cells. Cytology: Pap, 40×.

6.4. Differential Diagnosis of Normal Endometrial Cells

In table 6.1 we present the main cytological features distinguishing normal endometrial epithelial cells from stromal cells. In table 6.2 we compare the arrangement, size, nuclear features and cytoplasm of normal endometrial cells, endocervical cells and histiocytes (figs. 6.20, 6.21). It is not difficult to distinguish cells of secretory endometrium from endocervical cells.

Cytology of the Normal Endometrium –
Cycling and Postmenopausal

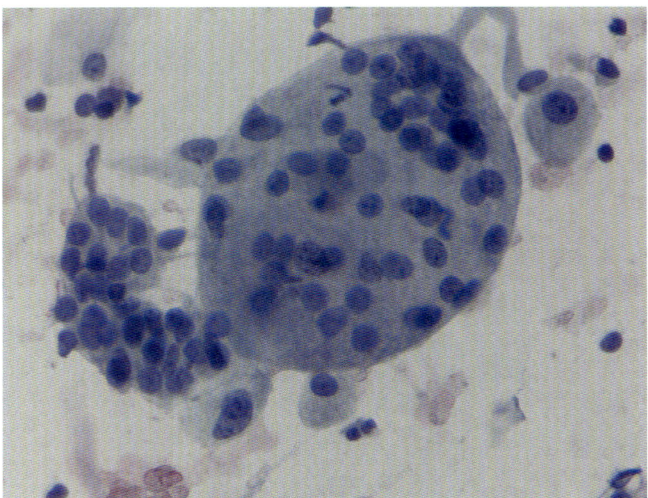

Fig. 6.21. Differential diagnosis with histiocytes. Pap, 40×.

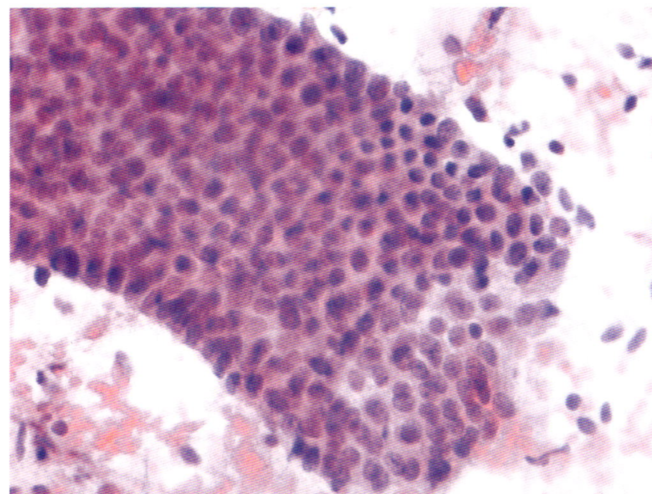

a

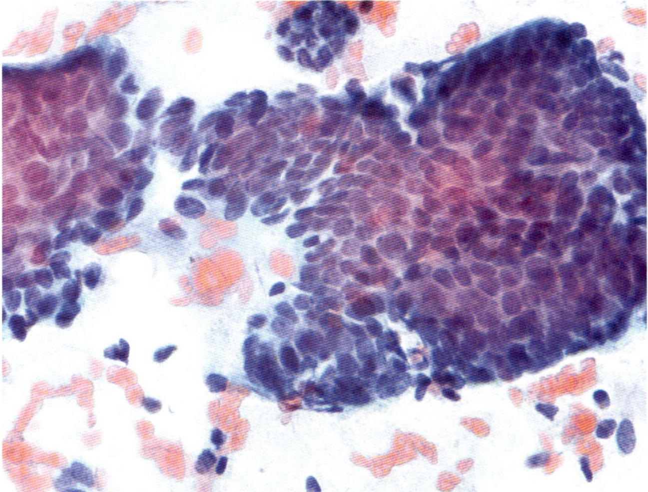

b

Fig. 6.22. Differential diagnosis of **a** late proliferative phase and **b** cystic hyperplasia. Endometrial brushing: 20×.

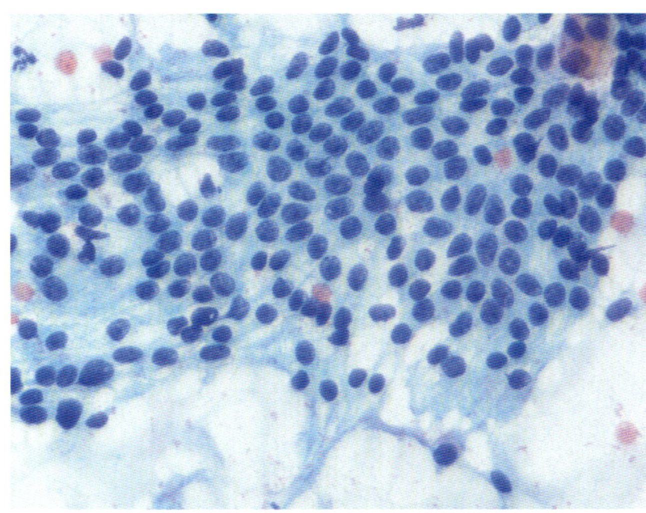

Fig. 6.23. Differential diagnosis of pseudodecidual cells with hyperplasia. Endometrial brushing: 40×.

We consider it useful to comment on some specific situations, which frequently present diagnostic problems in the routine examination of endometrial smears. To differentiate between proliferative and inactive endometrium, we must look carefully for mitotic figures, which are more frequent in a proliferative endometrium. It is more problematic to distinguish between late proliferative endometrium and cystic hyperplasia (fig. 6.22). Prominent overlapping of cells within sheets and increased number of mitoses is more evident in hyperplasia. Finally, pseudodecidual cells could be confused with cells of hyperplasia due to the irregular arrangement and overlapping of cells in the sheets. A careful evaluation of the cytoplasmic features and confirming the absence of mitoses will be useful (fig. 6.23).

Chapter 7

Benign Endometrial Lesions

While endometrial cytology has been widely recognized as a reliable technique in the diagnosis of premalignant and malignant lesions of the endometrium, very little has been published about benign endometrial lesions. The main reason may be the limitations of cytology in making a specific diagnosis of benign lesions and that a biopsy is therefore generally preferred. The cytological aspects of benign endometrial lesions are summarized in this chapter (table 7.1).

7.1. Inflammation

A diagnosis of endometritis depends on the presence of specific cellular components. Lymphocytes and poly-morphonuclear leukocytes are normally present in different phases of endometrial growth and maturation. In contrast, plasma cells are not normally present in the endometrium.

Except for rare forms of endometritis established by hematogenous implantation or descending infection from the fallopian tubes (e.g. tuberculosis), most types of endometritis result from ascending infection through the cervix, mainly during menses, abortion, delivery or instrumentation.

7.1.1. Non-Specific Acute and Chronic Endometritis
Acute endometritis is reflected in smears by a dirty background and an inflammatory infiltrate of neutrophils and lymphocytes. As in other inflammatory processes, epithelial cells may present reactive atypical changes, which can sometimes raise the differential diagnosis of malignancy. Moreover, acute endometritis may be associated with an endometrial cancer.

Chronic endometritis is associated with IUD, abortion or pregnancy, generally when the endometrium does not shed. It is characterized by a stromal inflammatory infiltrate of lymphocytes and plasma cells. The identification of plasma cells is regarded by many as the sine qua non of chronic endometritis (fig. 7.1).

7.1.2. Specific Endometritis
Tuberculosis. Tuberculous endometritis caused by *Mycobacterium tuberculosis* is a manifestation of a systemic

Table 7.1. Benign endometrial lesions

1. Inflammation
2. Dysfunctional uterine bleeding
3. Effects of radiation
4. Benign endometrial tumors: endometrial polyps

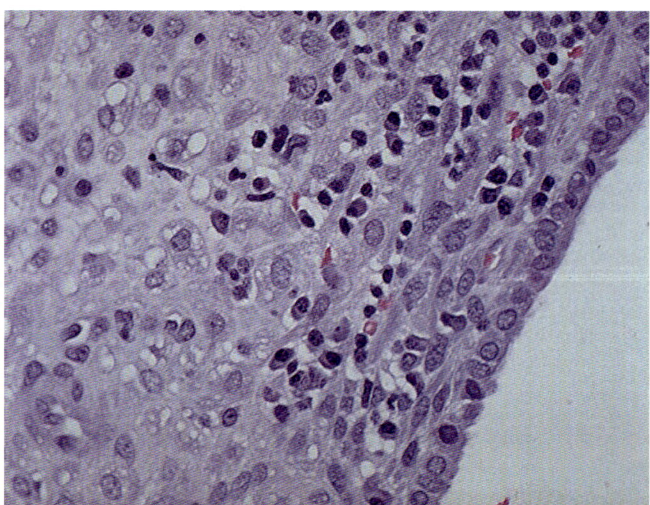

Fig. 7.1. Chronic endometritis. Presence of plasma cells. Histology: HE, 40×.

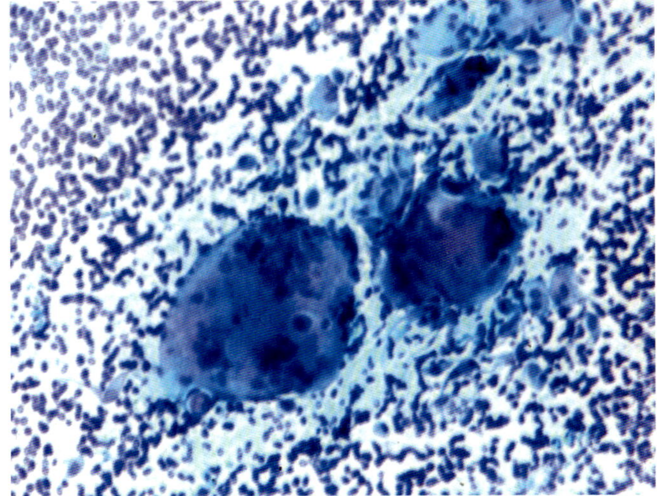 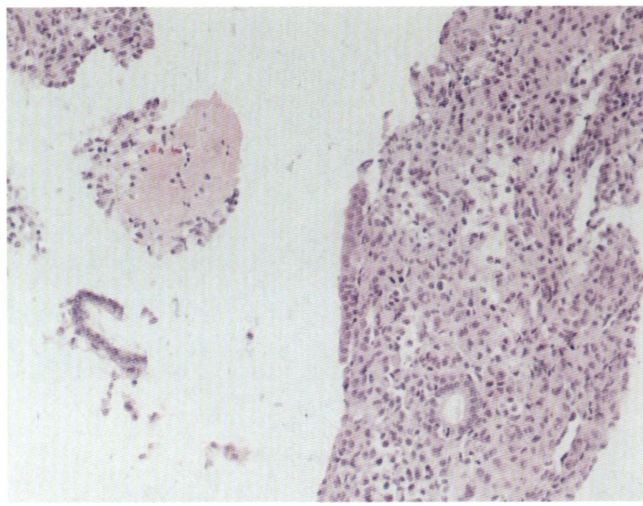

Fig. 7.2. Chronic inflammation with multinucleated histiocytes. Pap, 40×.

Fig. 7.3. Glandular and stromal breakdown. Cell block: HE, 20×.

disease. The endometrium is the second most commonly infected site in the female genital tract after the fallopian tubes. Patients with tuberculous endometritis are nearly always sterile because endometrial involvement develops secondarily from tubal infection.

The histological diagnosis of tuberculosis is difficult and there have been few reports of the cytological findings and diagnosis [164]. Typical granulomatous inflammation with Langhans giant cells is not always present, and a non-specific endometritis with lymphocytes and plasma cells may be the only manifestation (fig. 7.2). If tuberculosis is suspected, a curettage should be performed during the late secretory or menstrual phase of the cycle, before any granulomas possibly present are shed during the menses.

Fungal Infections. Rare infections by blastomycosis, coccidiomycosis, candida and crytococcosis have been described in histological reports. We have found no reports of the cytological diagnosis of fungal infections although it should be possible to demonstrate fungal elements in smears using special stains.

Viral Infections. Herpes virus, cytomegalovirus and human papillomavirus are the only viruses known to infect the endometrium. Ground-glass nuclei, round basophilic inclusions or koilocytes may respectively be found in cytological samples.

Parasitic Infections. Schistosoma, Enterobius vermicularis and *Echinococcus granulosus* present with a granulomatous inflammation simulating tuberculosis. *Toxoplasma gondii* produces a non-specific inflammation of the endometrium.

7.2. Dysfunctional Uterine Bleeding

Dysfunctional uterine bleeding (DUB) is a clinical term used to describe bleeding not attributable to an underlying organic pathologic condition. DUB generally results from derangement in the magnitude or duration of estrogen and progesterone effects on the endometrium.

Bleeding as a result of anovulatory cycles is the most common cause of DUB in women in the reproductive age group, but it characteristically occurs at menarche and at menopause. Histological examination shows glandular and stromal breakdown with proliferative glands and stromal cell condensation (fig. 7.3). In fact, it is a proliferative endometrium where the normal architecture has collapsed. As in other organs, cytology is limited when architectural criteria are the basis of the diagnosis. Furthermore, squamous, mucinous or ciliated metaplasias can occur, and special attention must be paid to eosinophilic syncytial change. In eosinophilic syncytial change, the cells have prominent eosinophilic cytoplasm and nuclei are enlarged, irregular and may present small nucleoli. This is not real atypia, and should not be misinterpreted. We must remember that anovulatory cycles are typical around menopause and present as bleeding, so our main differential diagnoses are pre-malignant and malignant lesions. These changes can be a real challenge in cytology, where glandular and stromal breakdown is difficult to diagnose without architectural criteria (figs. 7.4, 7.5).

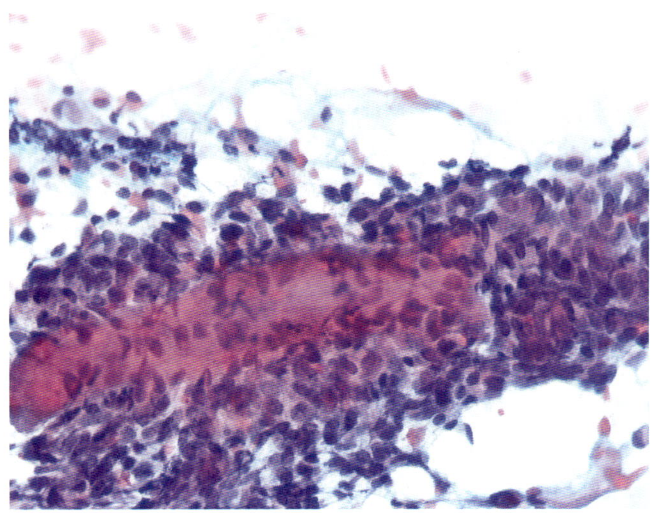

Fig. 7.4. Glandular and stromal breakdown. Disorganized endometrial group and a possible vessel or fibrin aggregate. Pap, 40×.

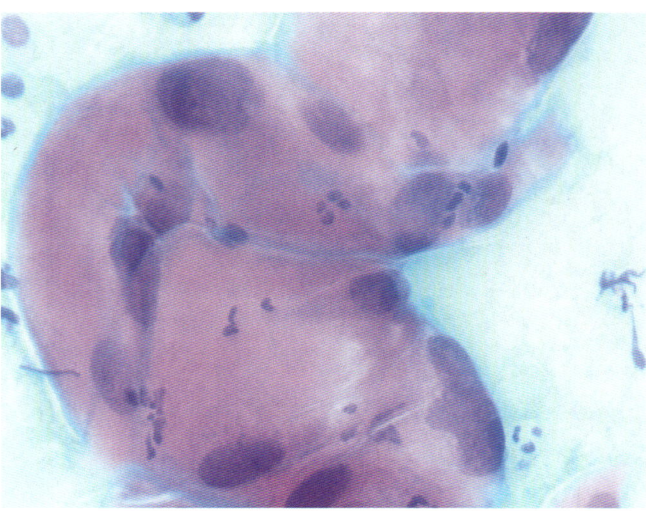

Fig. 7.6. Effects of radiation. Nuclear enlargement, pleomorphism and hyperchromasia and a large cytoplasm. Pap, 60×.

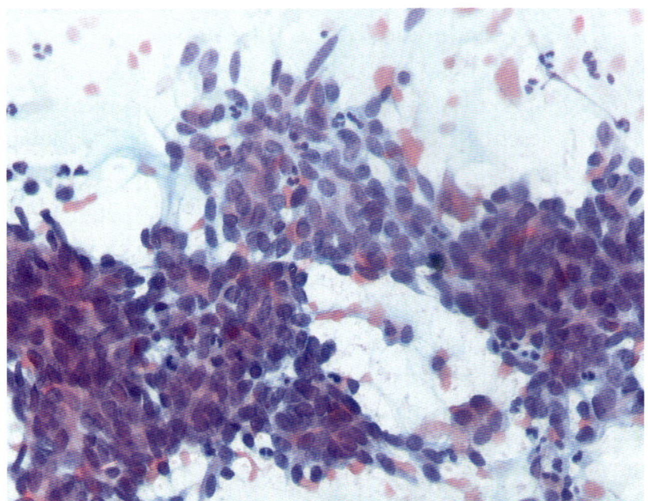

Fig. 7.5. Glandular and stromal breakdown. Presence of neutrophiles in a disorganized endometrial group. Pap, 40×.

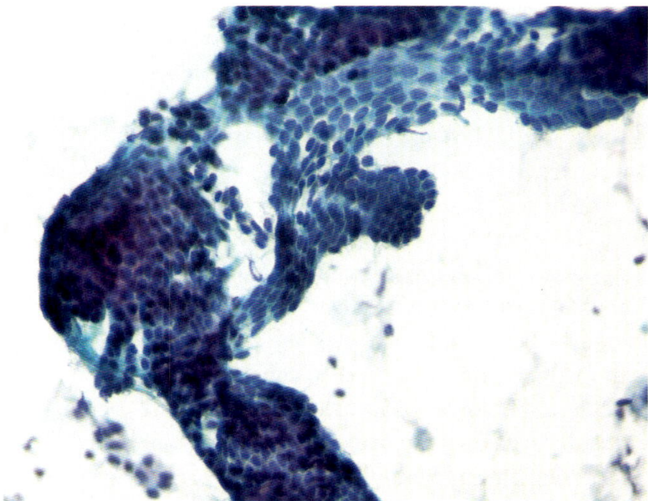

Fig. 7.7. Endometrial polyp. Large non-atypical epithelial sheet. Pap, 20×.

7.3. Effects of Radiation

As in other organs, radiation causes nuclear changes such as enlargement, pleomorphism and hyperchromasia (fig. 7.6). The cytoplasm often becomes granular and vacuolated. Postradiation changes can be difficult to differentiate from recurrent endometrial carcinoma.

7.4. Benign Endometrial Tumors

Endometrial polyps are by far the most frequent benign endometrial tumor. The prevalence of endometrial polyps in the general female population is estimated to be approximately 25% [187]. A higher prevalence of endometrial polyps is found among menopausal women treated with tamoxifen as

Benign Endometrial Lesions

well as in women with cervical polyps, in women of an advanced age and in those undergoing hormonal replacement therapy. Abnormal uterine bleeding is frequently the presenting symptom but polyps are often asymptomatic and found during routine ultrasound examination.

The endometrial polyp is a pedunculated or sessile excrescence of the endometrium containing variable amounts of glands, stroma and blood vessels. Histological diagnosis can be very difficult when the specimen is fragmented. In the same way, a specific cytological diagnosis is usually not possible. Endometrial cytology can rule out malignancy in many cases, but is not able to differentiate if the epithelium obtained is part of a polyp or from the surface of the endometrium (fig. 7.7).

Another point to bear in mind is the association of premalignant changes, and even carcinomas confined to polyps. In one study, the rate was high (6.3%) and old age, menopausal status and polyps >1.5 cm were associated with significant premalignant or malignant changes [9].

Chapter 8

Cytopathology of Endometrial Hyperplasias

8.1. Introduction

Endometrial hyperplasia (EH) is currently regarded as a spectrum of morphologic alterations ranging from benign changes induced by an abnormal hormonal environment to premalignant disease (WHO). It is also accepted that EH is the most important precursor of endometrial cancer (EC) and that it precedes neoplasia by several years. As a consequence, diagnosis and treatment of such premalignant lesions of the endometrium represent a major objective for EC prevention and a major challenge to cytopathologists, pathologists and gynecologists.

8.2. Histopathology

8.2.1. Criteria for Histological Typing

EH is generally divided into four different categories based on architectural and cytological characteristics. Hyperplasia is designated as simple or complex (adenomatous) depending on the degree of architectural complexity, and as EH (typical) (fig. 8.1) or atypical hyperplasia (AH) depending on the cytological features.

8.2.2. WHO Classification of Endometrial Hyperplasia

Classification. Using the WHO classification, it is possible to identify many precancerous lesions. However, this classification needs to be modified on the basis of current criteria, which we will discuss later (Hecht). Many classifications had been proposed prior to 1994 when the WHO adopted its current scheme (table 8.1). This is in principle based on an assessment of the presence or absence of cytological atypia. Reproducibility is poor with an interobserver kappa value of 0.3–0.47 [77]. Molecular data was not available at the time. However, it remains the best available classification.

Hyperplasia (EH) without Atypia. The histological pattern shows an excessive proliferative response to an unopposed estrogenic stimulus: the endometrium reacts in a diffuse manner with a balanced increase of both glands and stroma. In some areas glands appear cystically dilated, which

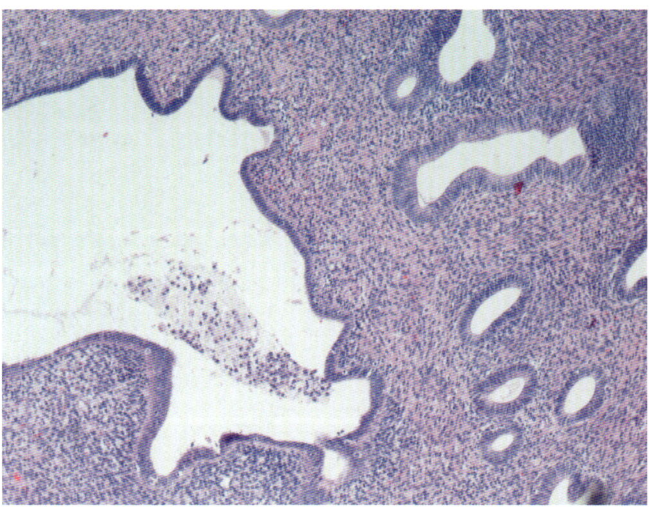

Fig. 8.1. Simple hyperplasia. Histology: HE, 10×.

Table 8.1. WHO classification of endometrial hyperplasia

Hyperplasia (typical)
– Simple hyperplasia without atypia
– Complex hyperplasia without atypia
  (adenomatous without atypia)

Atypical hyperplasia
– Simple
– Complex (adenomatous with atypia)

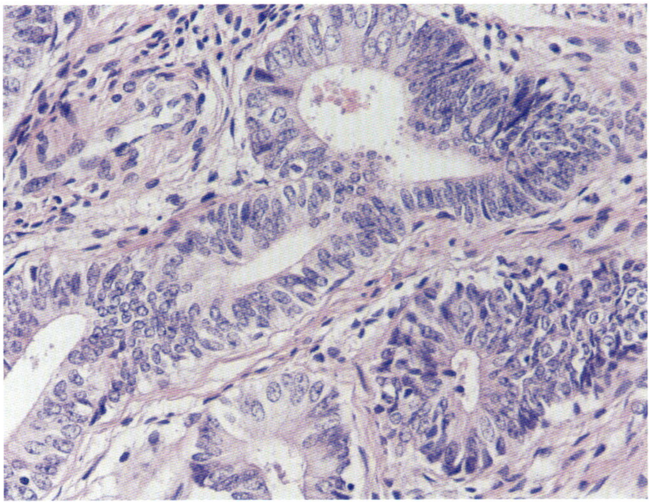

Fig. 8.2. Simple hyperplasia without atypia. Histology: HE, 40×.

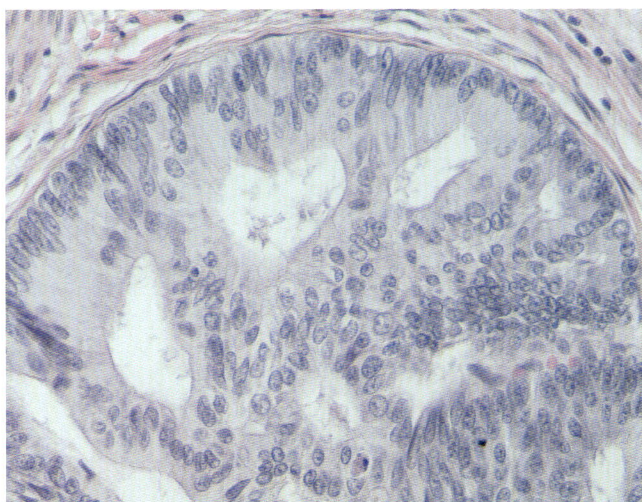

Fig. 8.3. Complex hyperplasia. Histology: HE, 40×.

contributes to an increase in the endometrial volume. The lining epithelium is pseudostratified to stratified, and its cells never show cytological atypia. They resemble those of proliferative endometrium. The glandular component may show a limited penetration into the stroma, and is sometimes active with occasional mitotic figures (fig. 8.2).

An important characteristic of EH without atypia is the low risk of progression to EC.

In simple hyperplasia, glands are tubular, frequently of a cystic or angular type, and their epithelial cells have elongated nuclei without atypia.

In complex hyperplasia (adenomatous without atypia) there is a greater degree of glandular proliferation and crowding, and architectural irregularity of size and shape of glands. Anarchic side buds and outpouching explain the typical 'finger in glove' appearance. Squamous epithelial morules may also be present. Cytological atypia is never present (fig. 8.3).

Atypical Endometrial Hyperplasia (AH). AH affects only the glands and not the stroma. It is usually focal but may be multifocal or diffuse. The glandular epithelium shows irregular stratification and loss of nuclear polarity. The reduced stroma causes the characteristic back-to-back arrangement of the glands. The key diagnostic features are the nuclear and cytoplasmic abnormalities of the glandular lining cells, in particular those seen in the nuclei; chromatin clearing, enlarged nucleoli and irregular nuclear membranes (fig. 8.4).

Simple AH is uncommon and shows the above features of atypical glandular cytology associated with the architecture of simple hyperplasia. In complex AH, there is both an increased glandular complexity and abnormal morphology with cytological atypia. Squamous morules are also

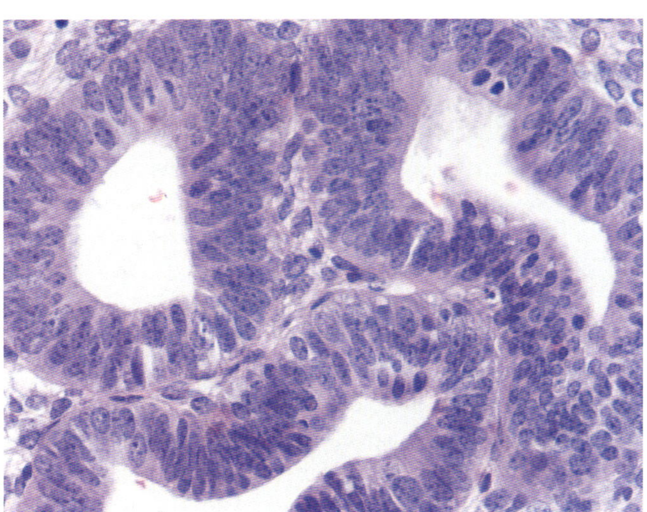

Fig. 8.4. Atypical hyperplasia. Histology: HE, 40×.

present. Evident features of adenocarcinoma (EA) are always absent.

AH is a premalignant disease with a high risk of progression to EC (approx. 30%) and requires more radical treatment than the EH.

8.2.3. Multicentric European Study on Endometrial Hyperplasia

The WHO classification of EH is generally accepted but the assessment of cytological atypia is a key problem in classifying individual cases into one of the four different WHO categories. When we try to separate the simple and the

Table 8.2. WHO classification European Pathologists' Classification (1999)

Proliferative endometrium Secretory endometrium Other	Cyclical endometrium
Simple hyperplasia Complex hyperplasia	Hyperplasia
Atypical hyperplasia Well-differentiated carcinoma	Endometrioid neoplasia

complex categories of EH without atypia we often find overlapping histological features of both processes [12]. In some cases it becomes difficult to decide what the crucial diagnostic feature is. Dietel [53] and other authors suggest that it may be preferable to consider only one category. Regardless of other considerations, both conditions need the same treatment with progestagens.

A similar situation occurs in relation to the simple and complex categories of AH. Besides, simple AH is almost non-existent. Finally, the distinction between AH and low-grade EC is often difficult.

A multicentric European study by five expert gynecological pathologists has been carried out to test the reproducibility of the WHO classification [12]. The intraobserver (85–89%) and interobserver (70–82%) agreements confirm that the difference between simple and complex hyperplasia is not reproducible. Both categories have the same prognosis and the distinction is not useful to clinicians either. It is preferable to assign both lesions to a single category named hyperplasia. The poor agreement in the histological diagnosis of complex hyperplasia and AH, and the lack of reproducibility in the histological recognition of stromal alteration to differentiate AH and well-differentiated EA suggest that the WHO classification should be simplified (table 8.2) when applied to biopsy and curettage specimens. This could be achieved by creating a combined category to include simple and complex hyperplasia called 'EH', and another combined category for AH and well-differentiated EA called 'endometrioid neoplasia' (EN) (figs. 8.5, 8.6) The European study found that the diagnoses of EH and EN were highly reproducible between observers from different institutions. Other important results of this study are that glandular crowding is the best histological feature to differentiate cyclical endometrium from EH, and that nuclear pleomorphism is the most reproducible cytological feature to differentiate EH from EN. The new term EN was introduced by Sherman and Brown [186]. Fox and Buckley [63] came to the same conclusion as the European pathologists.

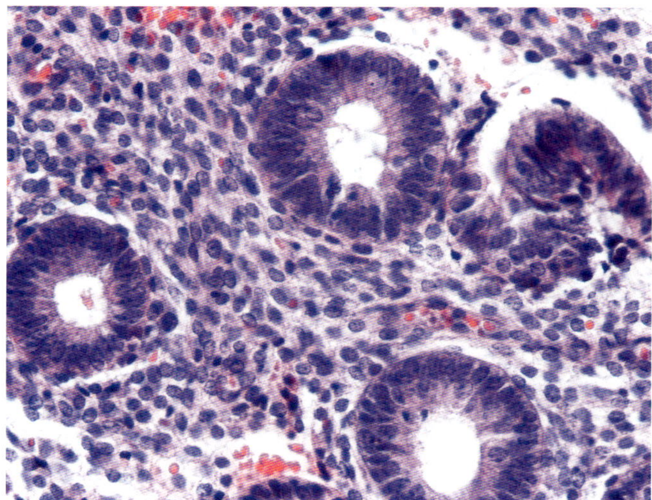

Fig. 8.5. Proliferative endometrium. Histology: HE, 40×.

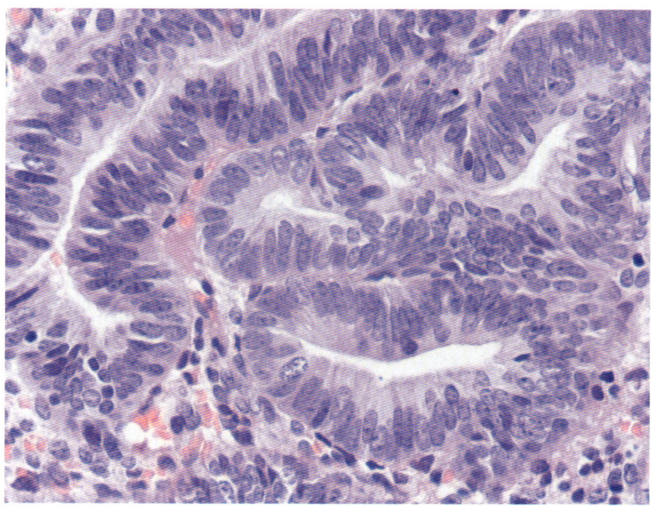

Fig. 8.6. Endometrioid neoplasia. Histology: HE, 40×.

8.2.4. Contemporary Approach to Endometrial Hyperplasia

The poor reproducibility of the 1994 WHO classification of EH is an important issue of debate. New concepts of pathogenesis of EH have been incorporated into an integrated genetic, histomorphometric and clinical outcome model of premalignant disease.

Following the European Multicentric Study (1999), a new approach has been proposed by Mutter [142] and the Endometrial Collaborative Group (ECG) (2000). This will be presented below. Both studies recommend a simplification of the WHO classification by reducing its four categories to two. This simplification has the advantage of a high degree

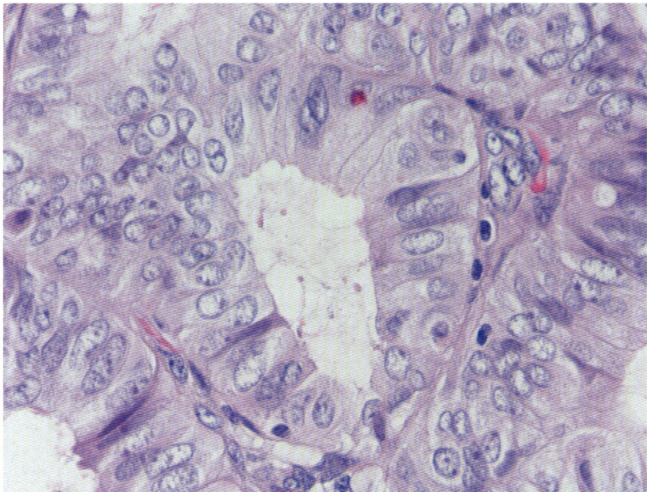

Fig. 8.7. Endometrial intraepithelial neoplasia. Histology: 60×.

Fig. 8.8. Well-differentiated endometrial adenocarcinoma. Histology: HE, 40×.

of reproducibility of histological diagnosis and facilitates the understanding by clinicians. Prognostic accuracy does not decrease. EH is a benign lesion easily treated by hormones with almost no risk of progression to EC. The second category (EN/EIN) is a premalignant or already malignant disease with a high risk of progression (about 30%), which needs more radical therapy [53].

Some authors [170, 192] do not agree with the new approach on endometrial intraepithelial neoplasia (EIN) but there is common agreement that the WHO classification needs to be modified [230]. The new classification of EIN and EN is gradually being accepted [191].

8.2.5. Endometrial Intraepithelial Neoplasia

Concept. Endometrial precancers are monoclonal benign neoplasms prone to malignant transformation. A type collection, organized by Mutter and the ECG, has identified precancers by their monoclonal growth and continuity of acquired genetic markers, which occur between premalignant and malignant phases of tumorigenesis. They call these premalignant lesions EIN, and have defined new architectural and cytological criteria using computerized morphometry [143].

Architectural Features. Four criteria must be met to diagnose a lesion as EIN: (1) the amount of glands exceed the amount of stroma with a reduction of stromal volume to less than half of the total sample volume; (2) epithelial cells within the architecturally abnormal focus must be cytologically different from those of the adjacent endometrium; (3) the size of the abnormal focus must exceed 1 mm, and (4) mimics of EIN and EC must be excluded (figs. 8.7, 8.8).

EIN Nomenclature Proposal for Endometrial Precancers. Mutter's proposed new classification (table 8.3) shows the diagnoses and the therapeutic implications of the new classification system of endometrial precancers using EIN terminology. Most AH according to the WHO nomenclature, and lesions with less atypical cytology but with an architectural pattern diagnostic of precancer, are focal and are considered to fall into the category of EIN. EH is generally diffuse. Anovulatory endometrium and endometrium exposed to unopposed estrogen is placed in the category of hyperplasia. Mutter [142] and the ECG as well as Koss and Melamed [106] suggest that monoclonaty and instability of microsatellites are the principal molecular abnormalities linking EIM to EC [77].

Hecht et al. [77] demonstrated a good correlation between subjectively applied criteria for the diagnosis of EIN and objective morphometry. They successfully segregated patients into high and low EC risk groups with better reproducibility (75% of cases) than a diagnosis of AH.

Management of EIN. This is quite similar to that previously offered to patients diagnosed as AH but can also include the option of hormonal therapy with progestin in conjunction with careful surveillance.

8.3. Cytopathology of Endometrial Hyperplasias

8.3.1. The Spanish Society of Cytology Endometrial Nomenclature

The nomenclature of the cytopathological patterns of endometrial lesions has been discussed by several institutions

Table 8.3. Data from Mutter et al. [142] and the Endometrial Collaborative Group (2000)

WHO nomenclature	EIN nomenclature	Functional category	Management
Simple nonatypical hyperplasia Complex nonatypical hyperplasia	EH, endometrial hyperplasia	Estrogen effect	Hormonal therapy
Simple atypical hyperplasia Complex atypical hyperplasia	EIN, endometrial intraepithelial neoplasia	Precancer	Hormonal or surgical therapy
Adenocarcinoma	Adenocarcinoma	Cancer	Based on stage

with a special interest in endometrial cytopathology. The Spanish Society of Cytology (SEC) [155], when recommending TBS for reporting vaginal and cervical cytology [112] to its members, extended the nomenclature to include endometrial cytology. The SEC included a category of cytological abnormalities (table 8.4) for which histological confirmation is recommended. The subtype 'atypical glandular cells' histologicallly corresponds to AH and well-differentiated EA. This is analogous to EN [9].

8.3.2. Current Status of Cytopathology of Endometrial Hyperplasias

No specific consideration of EH is given in TBS 2001. The only term used is 'atypical glandular cells (AGC)' if all cytological requirements for a diagnosis of glandular neoplasia are not fulfilled. Atypical glandular findings should be categorized as to cell type of origin (endocervical or endometrial). Cases of 'atypical endocervical cells' may be further qualified as 'favor neoplastic' but the smears of 'atypical endometrial cells' are not further qualified, reflecting the difficulty of subclassifying this category. As we mention in Chapter 2, atypical endometrial cells in smears may represent a major endometrial lesion such as EH, polyp (EP) or EA, but may also be related to chronic endometritis or IUD.

The Endometrial Forum of the TBS 2001 clarified that cervical cytology is primarily a screening test for squamous epithelial lesions and that it is unsuitable for the detection of endometrial lesions.

According to Meisels et al. [128] it is difficult to properly identify EH cytologically. They retrospectively reviewed 207 endometrial smears obtained by the Endopap endometrial sampler that had been histologically diagnosed as EH. Meisels found that five criteria provided an increased probability of correctly diagnosing EH in cytological samples: (1) the overlapping of cells in the glandular clusters or sheets; (2) the presence

Table 8.4. SEC endometrial nomenclature (1990)

Cell abnormalities/submit to histological confirmation:
– Atypical glandular cells (hyperplasia with cytological atypia well-differentiated adenocarcinoma)
– Glandular cells consistent with adenocarcinoma
– Cells consistent with sarcomas and other mesenchymal tumors

of nucleoli; (3) anisokaryosis; (4) granularity of chromatin, and (5) sheets of stromal cells.

EH was discussed in two sessions at the XV International Congress of Cytology, (Santiago de Chile, 2004). The histopathological patterns were presented by F. Nogales and Ch. Bergeron at the Satellite Symposium with the SLAP devoted to 'A Controversy on Endometrial Neoplastic Lesions' [89, 154]. We presented our classification of the cytology of EH (Antwerp, 2001) [93] at the same symposium and in the panel on 'Endometrial Adenocarcinoma – Prevention and Early Diagnosis' [94]. J. Whittaker and B. Knight presented their results on the cytopathological features of EH [222]. They found a cytological diagnosis of EH to be reproducible and reported a diagnostic accuracy of up to 95% for EC and 69.2% for EH.

Noritmatsu et al. [156] have recently published interesting results using an Endocyte sampler device. They propose new diagnostic criteria based on the composition and architecture of tissue fragments. Cell aggregates with a tube or sheet-shaped pattern were found in 97.5% of samples of normal proliferative endometrium. In EH, cell aggregates with a dilated or branched pattern were found in 34.9% of cases. Cell aggregates with irregular protrusions were seen in 61.8% of grade 1 EA, and a papillotubular pattern in 29.7% of cases. They also found that papillary metaplastic changes that contain condensed stromal clusters help to distinguish an anovulatory menstrual cycle from EH.

Cytopathology of Endometrial Hyperplasias

Table 8.5. Cytopathology of endometrial hyperplasia: Jiménez-Ayala classification (2001) (WHO: simple and complex)

Arrangement
– Regular
– Large widened glands, cell clusters and fragments
Cells
– Somewhat large
Nuclei
– Slight atypia. Uniform
– Chromatin finely dispersed
– Smooth membrane
– Micronucleoli
Background
– Absence of mitotic figures and tumor diathesis

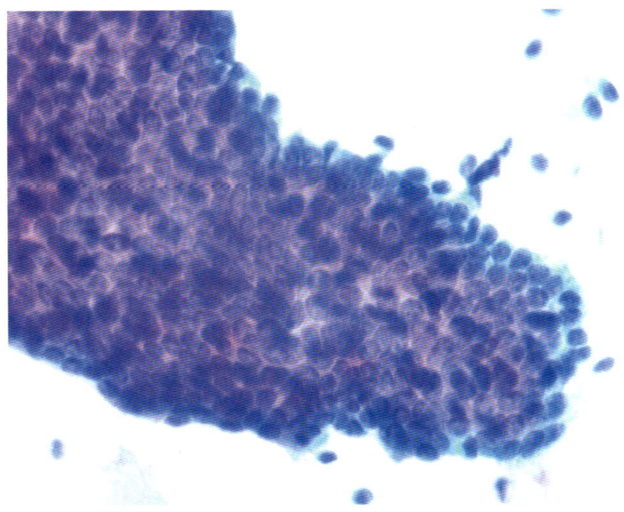

Fig. 8.9. Cytology of endometrial hyperplasia. Large endometrial cells with loss of regular arrangement. Pap, 40×.

8.3.3. Practical Considerations in the Cytopathology of Endometrial Hyperplasia

It is clear from the observations discussed above that specific endometrial sampling techniques must be used to adequately assess the cytopathology of endometrial lesions. Among the different techniques described in Chapter 3, endometrial brushing techniques give the highest accuracy. Furthermore, after 35 years' experience of endometrial cytopathology, we concluded that a pragmatic classification was needed. We first presented our classification, modified from the European Pathologists' Classification, at the XIV International Congress of Cytology (Amsterdam, 2001) [93].

8.4. Cytopathology of Endometrial Hyperplasias. The Jiménez-Ayala Classification

Endometrial Hyperplasia (table 8.5)

We found that the simple and complex hyperplasia of the WHO classification present the same cytological pattern, as was also reported by Nguyen and Kline [151]. The material obtained by endometrial brushing techniques is abundant showing a regular pattern of large, widened glands, cell clusters [135] and fragments of sheets (figs. 8.9, 8.12). Coscia-Porrazzi [41] found dilated and branching glandular structures in cellular sheets in complex hyperplasia, resembling the histological features of adenomatous hyperplasia. Ohno [160] reported that large rounded and ball-like aggregates facilitate the diagnosis.

The epithelial cells are large and show slight nuclear atypia but a uniform, finely dispersed, or sometimes, dense chromatin, with smooth nuclear membranes and frequent micronucleoli (figs. 8.10, 8.11, 8.13). Tumoral diathesis and mitotic figures are absent in the smears.

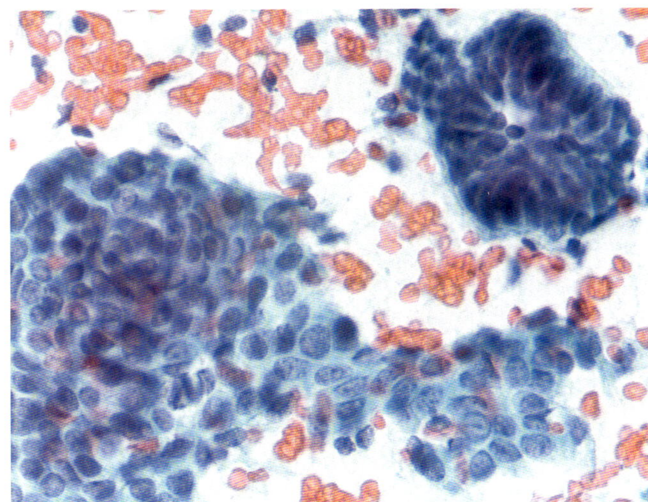

Fig. 8.10. Endometrial hyperplasia. Nuclei with finely dispersed chromatin and small nucleoli. Pap, 40×.

Endometrioid Neoplasia (table 8.6)

In accordance with the histopathological concept of the European Pathologists' Classification, we include in this category the cytopathological features of AH and of well-differentiated EA (fig. 8.14). Endometrial brushing techniques show large sheets and clusters of overlapping and pleomorphic cells (fig. 8.15). The pleomorphism is, as in histological sections, the main feature that differentiates between EH and EN. The cells in three-dimensional clusters are large with enlarged, crowded and well-defined pleomorphic

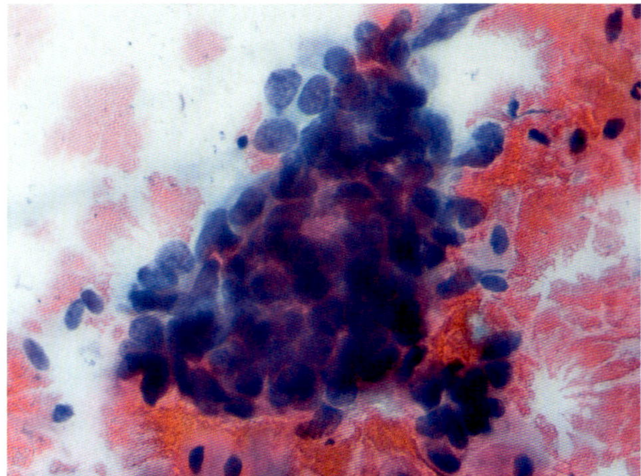

Fig. 8.11. Endometrial hyperplasia. Hyperchromasia and coarse chromatin. Pap, 60×.

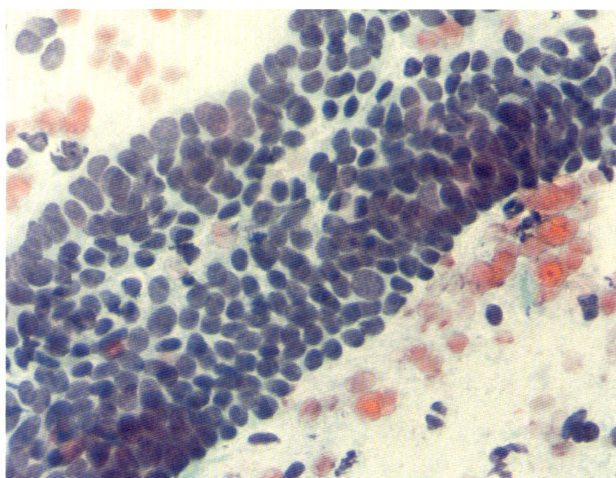

Fig. 8.12. Endometrial hyperplasia. Large cell clusters. Pap, 40×.

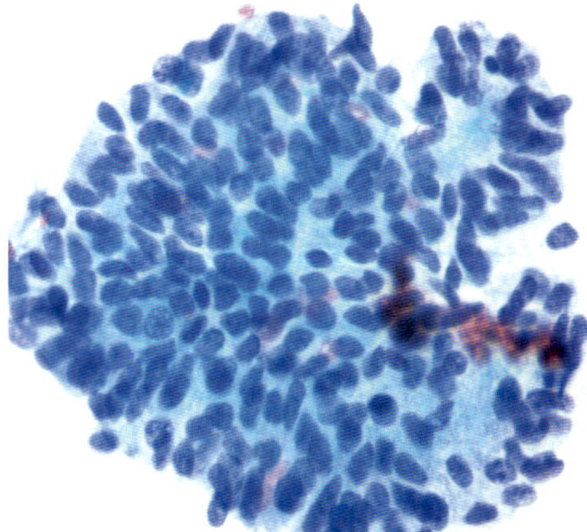

Fig. 8.13. Endometrial hyperplasia. Granular chromatin and small nucleoli. Pap, 40×.

Table 8.6. Cytopathology of endometrial hyperplasia: Jiménez-Ayala classification (2001) (WHO: atypical hyperplasia and well-differentiated adenocarcinoma)

Arrangement
– Large sheets and clusters: three-dimensional
– Overlapping and pleomorphic

Cells
– Large and pleomorphic

Nuclei
– Large and pleomorphic
– Crowding and parachromatin clearing
– Uneven border
– Coarse chromatin
– Nucleoli: small and medium size

Stroma
– Large clusters
– Pale pleomorphic cells
– Oval nuclei
– Ill-defined cytoplasm

Background
– Absent or scarce tumoral necrosis

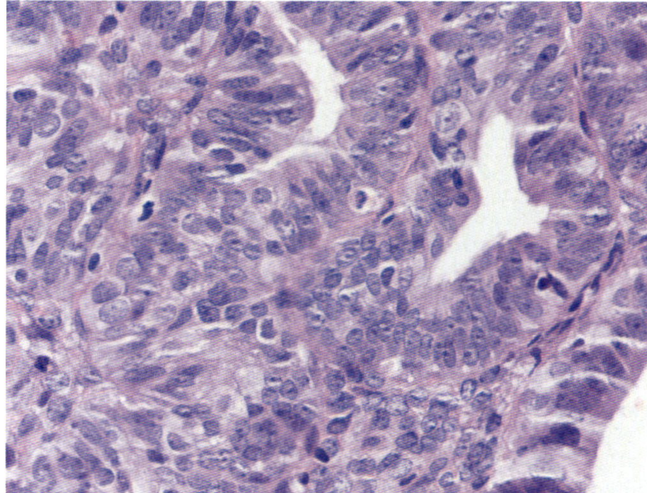

Fig. 8.14. Endometrioid neoplasia. Histology: HE, 40×.

nuclei (fig. 8.16). The nuclear chromatin is coarse, nuclear borders are uneven and there are small and medium-sized nucleoli (figs. 8.17, 8.18), contrasting with the nuclei of cells of EH.

The presence of large clusters of lightly pleomorphic stromal cells with oval nuclei and ill-defined cytoplasm [150] help in the diagnosis. Tumoral necrosis in the smear background is absent or minimal (fig. 8.19).

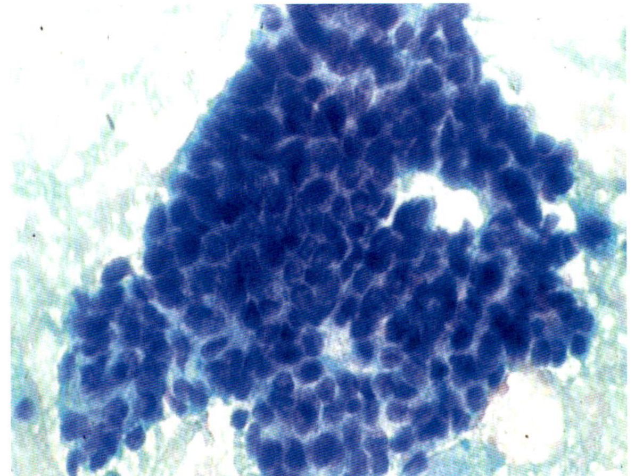

Fig. 8.15. Endometrioid neoplasia. Overlapping and three-dimensional groups. Pap, 60×.

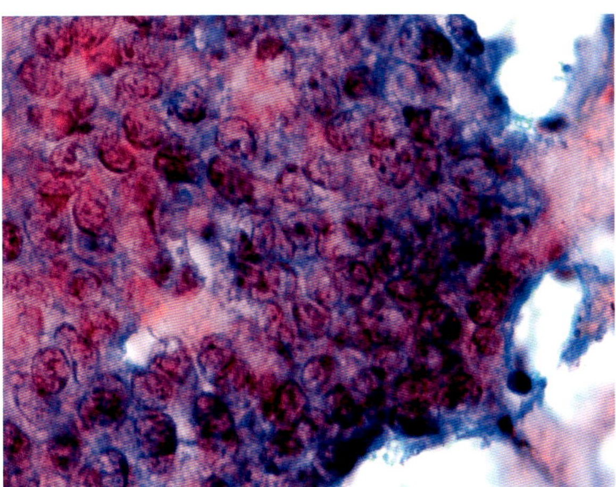

Fig. 8.18. Endometrioid neoplasia. Uneven nuclei with medium-sized nucleoli. Pap, 60×.

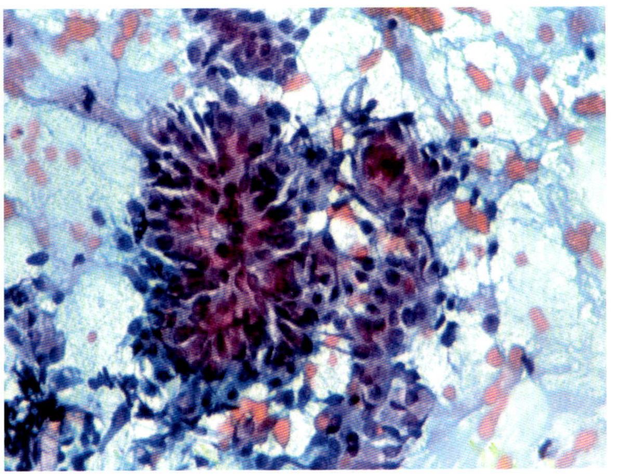

Fig. 8.16. Endometrioid neoplasia. Hyperchromatic and pleomorphic nuclei. Pap, 40×.

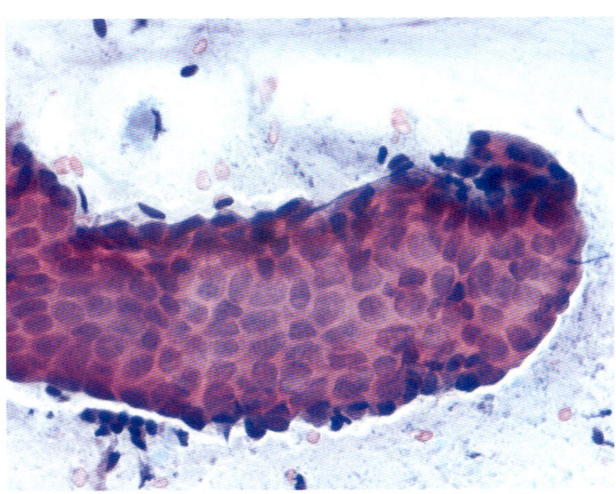

Fig. 8.19. Endometrioid neoplasia. Pleomorphic cells with minimal necrosis. Pap, 40×.

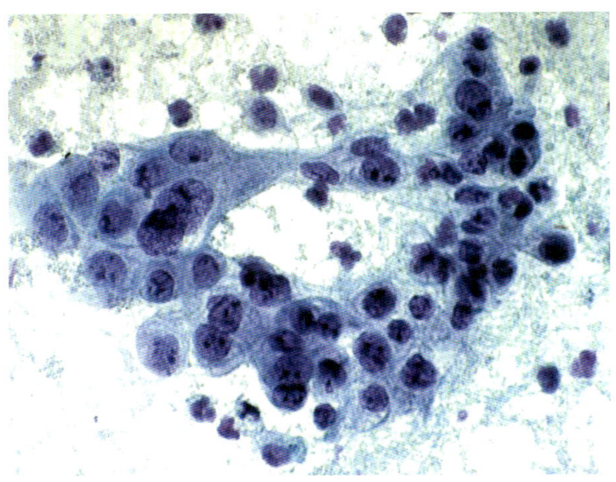

Fig. 8.17. Endometrioid neoplasia. Cytology. Coarse chromatin and nucleoli. Pap, 60×.

Final Remarks and Conclusions

We propose that the Jiménez-Ayala classification of the cytopathology of endometrial hyperplasia is based on current concepts of the pathology of EH and that it meets the requirements for a classification of the precursors of EC.

Chapter 9

Cytopathology of Endometrial Adenocarcinoma

9.1. Problems and Accuracy for the Cytological Diagnosis of Endometrial Adenocarcinoma

Problems

As we pointed out in Chapter 1, the cervicovaginal smear (CVS) is not particularly efficient at detecting endometrial adenocarcinoma (EA). Endometrial brushing techniques (EBT) are therefore necessary. The main reasons for the low accuracy of the Pap are as follows: (1) EA usually desquamates sparsely producing scanty and inconsistent samples. (2) There may be obstacles to CVS such as cervical stenosis and synechia, endocervical polyps, submucous myoma or vaginal cleisis. (3) In some cases, EA extends mainly into the myometrium. (4) Degeneration of cells during the passage from the endometrial cavity to the posterior vaginal vault. (5) The posterior vaginal vault has not been sampled. (6) Interpretative difficulties: distinction from endometrial hyperplasia (EH).

Accuracy

The accuracy of cytological diagnosis of EA depends on several factors, intrinsic or extrinsic. Intrinsic factors are host factors or tumor-related factors such as anatomical localization, morphologic type and grade of differentiation. Extrinsic factors are types of sampling (CVS or EBT), and training and specific experience in endometrial cytopathology of the laboratory staff (cytopathologists and cytotechnologists).

9.2. Classification of Endometrial Epithelial Tumors

The different types of endometrial epithelial tumors included in the 2003 WHO histological classification of tumors of the uterine corpus are presented in table 9.1.

Adenocarcinoma in situ was not included because adequate cytologic criteria for this diagnosis do no exist. This chapter is devoted to the cytopathological features of EA and to the less common types of cancers, preceded by a basic description of their histopathology and by some comments on the clinical aspects.

Clinical Features of EA. EA is a tumor predominantly of postmenopausal women with a peak incidence between 50 and 60. It most commonly presents with postmenopausal bleeding. In the few patients younger than 40, the most common clinical sign is menometrorrhagia. The histological type is EA in about 80–85% of cases, a low-grade, estrogen-dependent tumor. The patients are frequently obese, diabetic, infertile, or have a late menopause. It is important to remember that patients with EH and atypical hyperplasia have similar clinical associations (WHO). The mucinous type of EA also has similar features and prognosis. In contrast, the non-estrogen-dependent tumors including papillary serous,

Table 9.1. Epithelial tumors of the uterine corpus (WHO, 2003)

Endometrial carcinoma:
– Endometrioid adenocarcinoma
    Variant with squamous differentiation
    Villoglandular variant
    Secretory variant
    Ciliated cell variant
– Mucinous adenocarcinoma
– Serous adenocarcinoma
– Clear cell adenocarcinoma
– Mixed cell adenocarcinoma
– Squamous cell carcinoma
– Small cell carcinoma
– Undifferentiated carcinoma
– Others

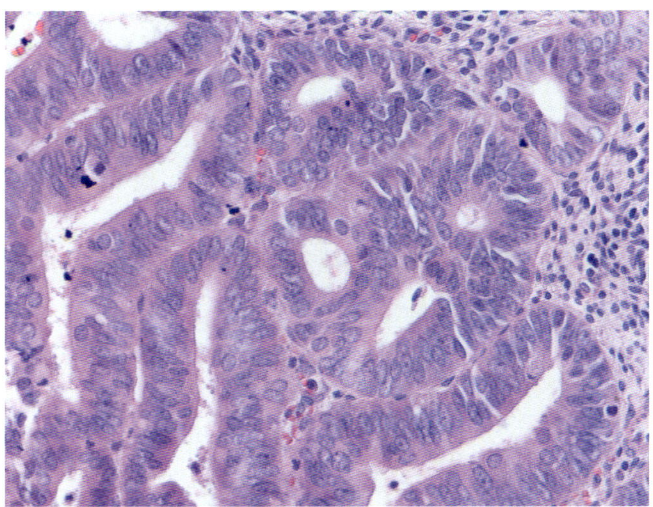

Fig. 9.1. Histopathology of endometrioid adenocarcinoma. Histology: HE, 40×.

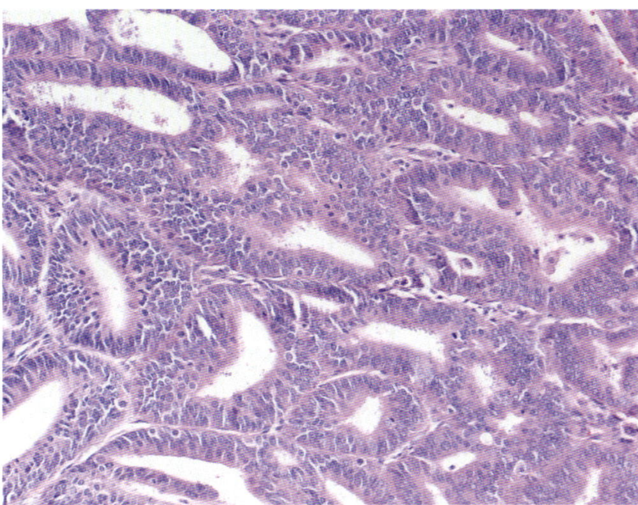

Fig. 9.2. Endometrioid adenocarcinoma grade 1. Histology: HE, 20×.

clear-cell and adenosquamous carcinomas, are in a more advanced stage at diagnosis and have a worse prognosis [31].

9.3. Histopathology of Endometrioid Adenocarcinoma

Concept. An EA, the glands of which resemble those of normal endometrium (fig. 9.1). Endometrioid adenocarcinoma (EnA) accounts for approximately 90% of EA [32]. These tumors are usually primary in the endometrium, but may also develop in endometrial polyps (EP) and in foci of endometriosis that may be located in a variety of sites including the ovary [106].

Microscopic Features. EnA shows a spectrum of patterns varying from very well-differentiated carcinoma to poorly-differentiated tumor, which is the basis of the histological grading described below.

EnA typically has tubular glands, mostly of medium size. The glands are usually round to oval, but they are sometimes angulated or branching. Associated with the glands is a variable amount of endometrial stroma. The neoplastic glands are lined by stratified or pseudostratified columnar cells with rounded nuclei, prominent nucleoli and scanty eosinophilic cytoplasm. Necrosis of glands and necrotic debris are common in poorly-differentiated adenocarcinoma. Coexistent EH is present in 18–45% of EnA [32, 162].

Grading of EnA. The prognostic relevance of grading EnA has been recognized for many years. The most widely accepted grading system is the 1988 FIGO/ISGP with modifications

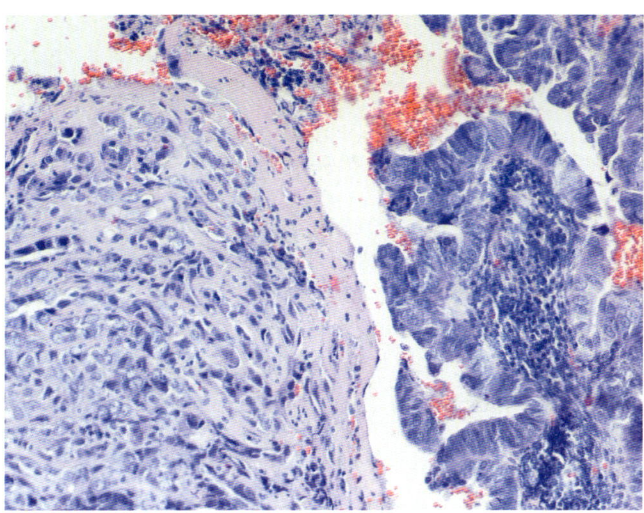

Fig. 9.3. Moderately-differentiated, grade 2, endometrioid adenocarcinoma. Histology: HE, 20×.

suggested by Zaino [231] who classified EnA by architectural and nuclear features. The main details of this grading are summarized as follows:

Grade 1 or well-differentiated: Tumors are <5% solid with a cribiform pattern of dilated glands, prominent nuclear atypia and mitotic activity (fig. 9.2).

Grade 2 or moderately-differentiated carcinomas: The glands are smaller with a predominantly cribiform continuous pattern resembling a garland. 5–50% of the tumor tissue consists of solid areas (fig. 9.3).

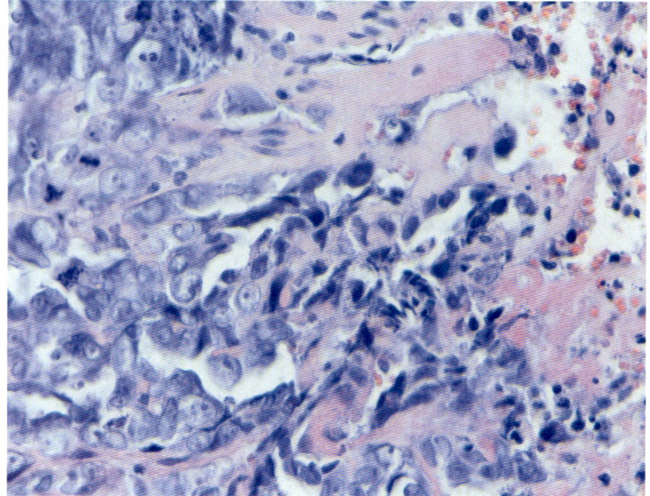

Fig. 9.4. Poorly-differentiated, grade 3, endometrioid adenocarcinoma. Histology: HE, 40×.

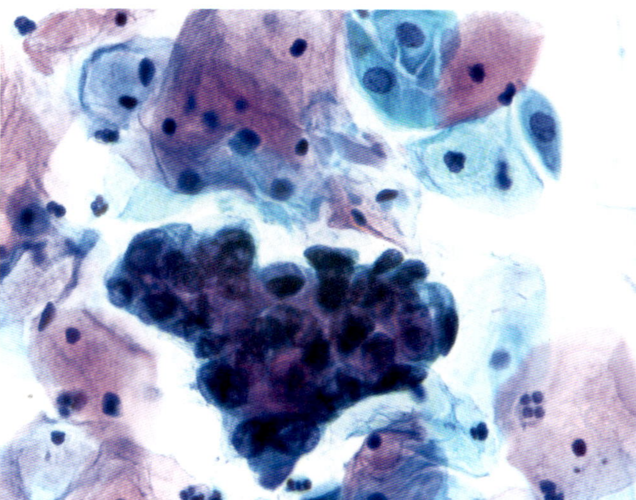

Fig. 9.5. Low-grade adenocarcinoma (CVS). Pap, 60×.

Grade 3 or poorly-differentiated: Tumors are solid to >50% with few glands and have an anaplastic appearance [32, 95, 97] (fig. 9.4).

Immunohistochemistry of Endometrioid Adenocarcinoma

EnA has a highly characteristic immunophenotype with coexpression of cytokeratin and vimentin and a focal high molecular weight cytokeratin expression. The investigation of estrogen and progesterone receptors and of the expression of p53 is very useful in the diagnosis of this tumor, and also in prognostication [228]. Serial CA-125 assay is a good indicator of disease activity and a useful biochemical tool for posttreatment surveillance of patients with EA [66].

An interesting cytologic scoring of EA has recently been published by Nishimura et al. [152] using endometrial smears. A high cytologic score was correlated with p53 mutation and myometrial invasion, and correlated negatively with estrogen and progesterone receptor status.

9.4. Cytopathological Grading of EnA

For practical cytodiagnostic and prognostic purposes it is commonly accepted that EnA can cytologically be divided into two grades or types [95]:

Low-grade carcinoma (well-differentiated) (fig. 9.5)
Shedding
–Three-dimensional papillary cell aggregates with peripheral nuclei

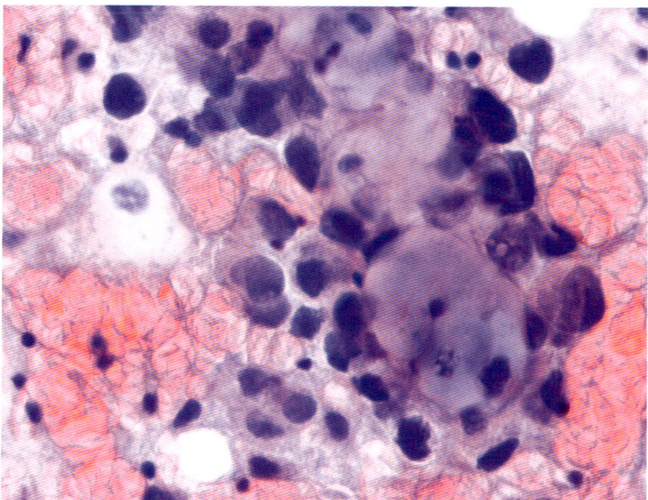

Fig. 9.6. High-grade adenocarcinoma. Endometrial smear. Pap, 60×.

– Cell aggregates forming 'rosettes' and glandular tubes
– Isolated cells
Malignant cells
– Stratification of tumor cells with nuclear crowding
– Anisokaryosis
– Micronucleoli. Few prominent nucleoli
Background
– Tumor diathesis absent or scanty. Fibroblast-like stromal cells and foamy cells
High-grade carcinoma (poorly-differentiated) (fig. 9.6)
Shedding

Cytopathology of Endometrial
Adenocarcinoma

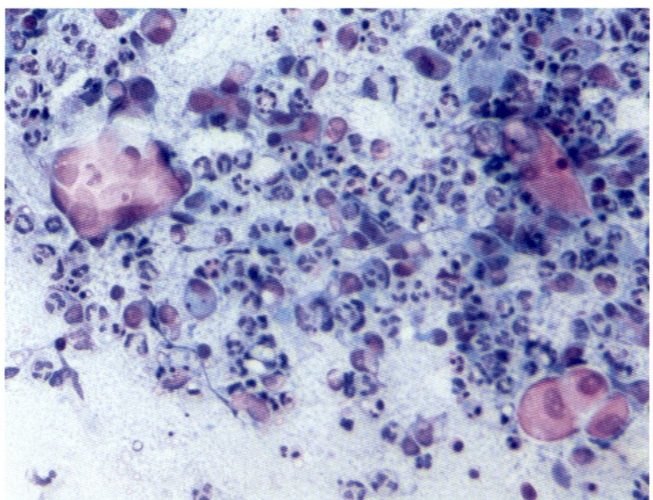

Fig. 9.7. Endometrioid adenocarcinoma. Advanced stage (CVS). Pap, 40×.

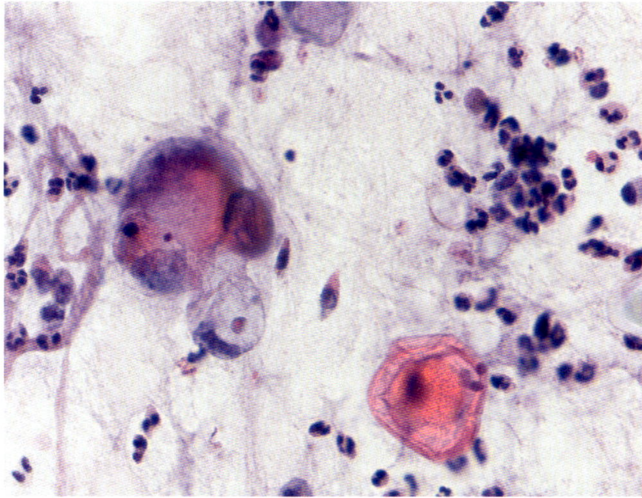

Fig. 9.8. Endometrial adenocarcinoma. Advanced stage (CVS). Pap, 60×.

Table 9.2. Endometrioid adenocarcinoma

Cytological features in CVS. Advanced stage:
- Patient is symptomatic
- Background: red blood cells and debris
- Microarchitecture: papillary grouping, sheets and rosettes
- Cytoplasm: finely vacuolated, signet-ring cells
- Nuclei: variable nucleoli, grossly abnormal chromatin

- Solid sheets and loose clusters of tumor cells
- Fewer papillary structures

Malignant cells
- Pleomorphic and bizarre glandular cells
- Cells larger than in low-grade carcinoma
- High nuclear/cytoplasmic ratio
- Irregular nuclear chromatin. Macronucleoli. Mitotic figures

Tumor background
- Necrotic debris and foamy histiocytes

9.5. Cytological Diagnosis of Endometrioid Adenocarcinoma

Cervicovaginal Smear

Although the accuracy of the CVS in detecting EnA is low, it can provide some useful information. Unfortunately, consistent cytological features usually only appear in an advanced stage when the patient presents with suspected postmenopausal bleeding. The main signs that permit a late cytological diagnosis are listed in table 9.2 (figs 9.7, 9.8).

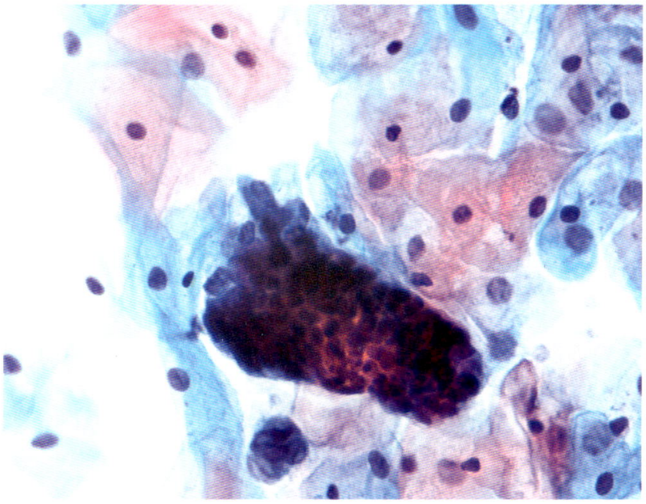

Fig. 9.9. Endometrial adenocarcinoma. Early stage (CVS). Pap, 40×.

Table 9.3. Endometrioid adenocarcinoma

Cytological features in CVS. Early stage:
- Few malignant cells
- Nuclei: granular chromatin and areas of chromatin clearing
- Prominent nucleoli

The percentage of nuclei with nucleoli and the size and number of nuclei in each nucleus are related to the histological type and grade of the tumor.

In a small number of cases it may be possible to make a cytological diagnosis at an early stage (table 9.3, fig. 9.9).

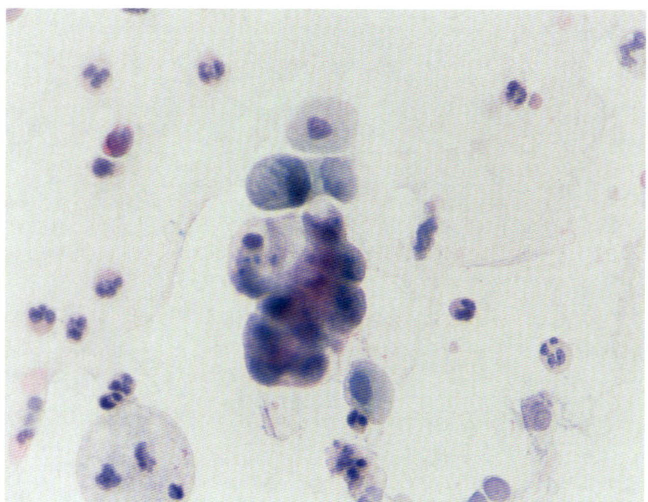

Fig. 9.10. Endomtrial cells in a 45-year-old patient on day 20 of the menstrual cycle can be a sign of possible endometrial pathology. Pap, 60×.

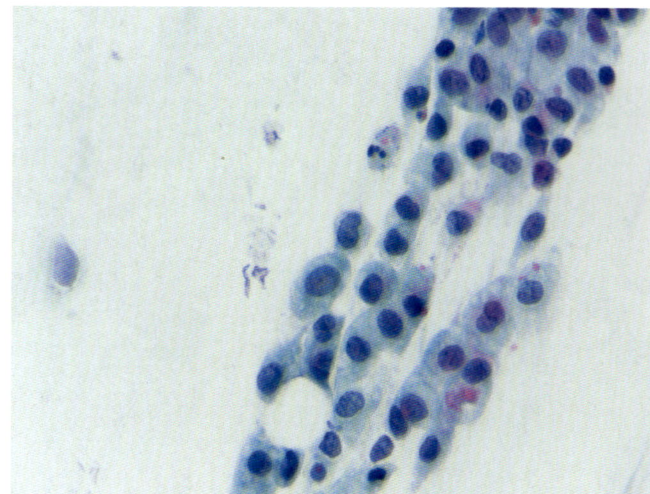

Fig. 9.11. Histocytes in CVS of postmenopausal woman. Pap, 60×.

Table 9.4. Endometrioid adenocarcinoma

Cytological features in CVS. Indirect signs:
– Normal endometrial cells
– Bloody background
– Small histiocytes
– Elevated estrogen effect

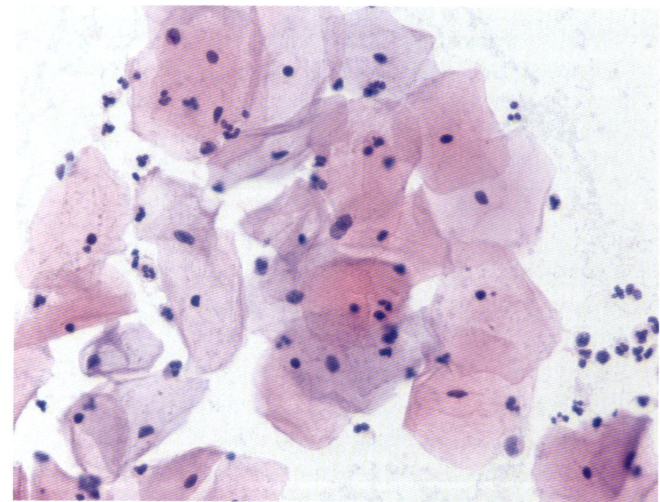

Fig. 9.12. Elevated estrogenic effect in postmenopausal patient (CVS). Pap, 40×.

Papanicolaou pointed to the presence of phagocytosed neutrophils in the vacuolized cytoplasm of glandular cells as a helpful sign. The significance of some indirect signs pointing to a cytological diagnosis of EA is a controversial subject (table 9.4). The Forum of EC of the 2001 Bethesda Conference recommended that the finding of normal endometrial cells in smears justified looking for potential endometrial pathology only in women over 40 years of age [197]. Our experience, and that of other authors [129], leads us to recommend EBT in women in whom a Pap has identified normal endometrial cells after the 12th day of the menstrual cycle, provided that the patient does not have an IUD (fig. 9.10). In the presence of an IUD, endometrial cells may be shed on the 15th day or later. We also consider that the presence of small histiocytes in the vaginal pool with no signs of infection, especially if associated with other indirect signs of possible tumor diathesis such as fresh blood or red-yellow blood, could make further investigation worthwhile (fig. 9.11).

Finally, an elevated estrogen effect in a postmenopausal woman not using hormone replacement therapy could be an indirect sign of a well-differentiated tumor (fig. 9.12). Smears are atrophic in cases with poorly-differentiated tumors.

Endometrial Brushing

The patterns of neoplastic shedding seen in EBT are shown in table 9.5. The cells form sheets, papillae (fig. 9.13) and rosettes. Although the cells are enlarged, the reduced

Cytopathology of Endometrial
Adenocarcinoma

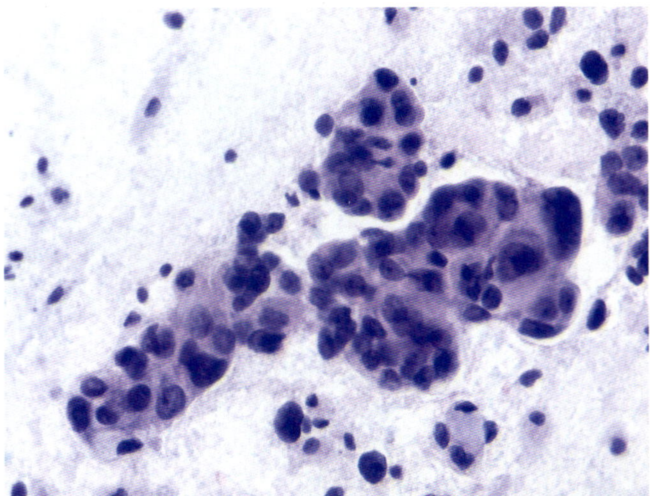

Fig. 9.13. Papillae in endometrial adenocarcinoma. Endometrial brushing. Pap, 60×.

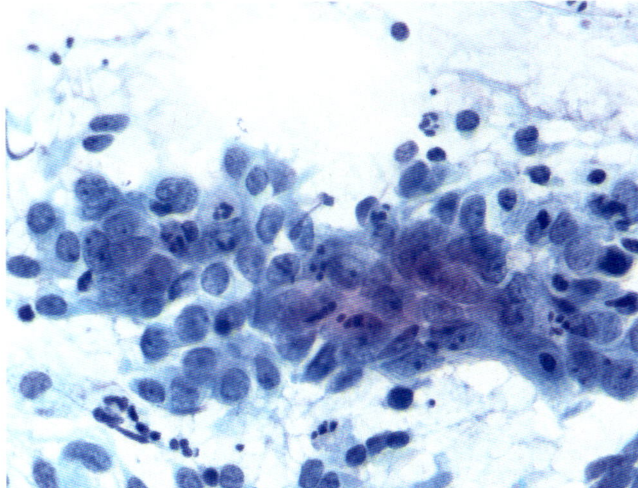

Fig. 9.14. Nuclear anomalies in endometrial adenocarcinoma. Pap, 60×.

Table 9.5. Endometrioid adenocarcinoma

Brushing technique. Endometrial shedding:
– Sheets
Loss of cell cohesion
Overlapping of cells
Cellular and nuclear polarity poorly preserved
– Arrangement
Papillae
Rosettes
Irregular sheets, enlarged cells
– Nuclei
Increased variation in size
Grossly irregular and reticular chromatin
Irregular nuclear membranes
Prominent and irregular nucleoli
– Cytoplasm
Variable amount
Atypical vacuolization
– Background
Tumor diathesis
Inflammation

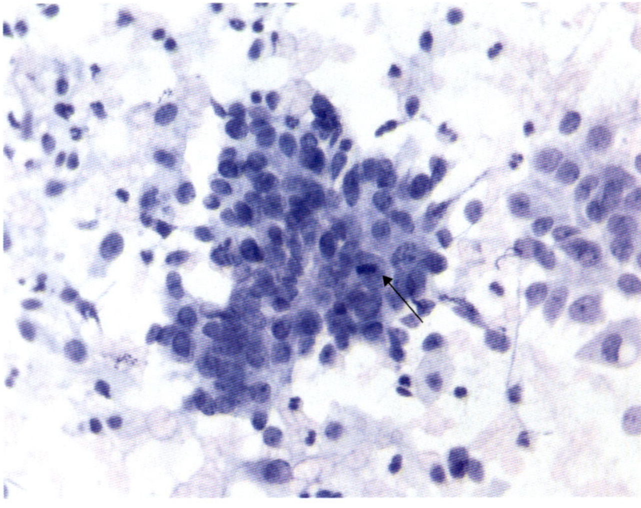

Fig. 9.15. Mitotic figure in endometrial brushing of endometrial adenocarcinoma. Pap, 40×.

amount of cytoplasm reverses the nuclear/cytoplasmic ratio. The periphery of the cell aggregates has an irregular tree branching-like appearance. The stromal cells are rarely seen as tissue fragments [160].

The nuclear features also listed in table 9.5 include margination of the chromatin which causes the appearance of areas of clearing (fig. 9.14). Mitotic figures are occasionally found (fig. 9.15). The amount of cytoplasm is variable. Most of the cells are reduced in size due to autolysis resulting in poorly-defined cell borders. Cytoplasmic vacuoles are of variable size and sometimes produce typical signet-ring cells (fig. 9.16). Finally there is necrotic debris associated with neutrophils, red blood cells and histiocytes in the background of smears from EA (fig. 9.17). Tumor diathesis may be scarce without fresh blood in patients with focal tumor. Clinical pyometra in older patients causes degeneration of neoplastic cells that render the differential diagnosis of acute endometritis difficult. Any smear looking like endometritis in a postmenopausal woman is a priori suspected of malignancy [115].

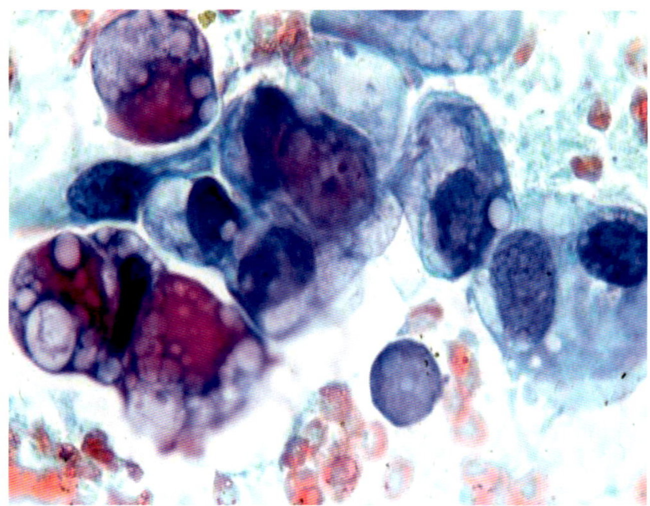

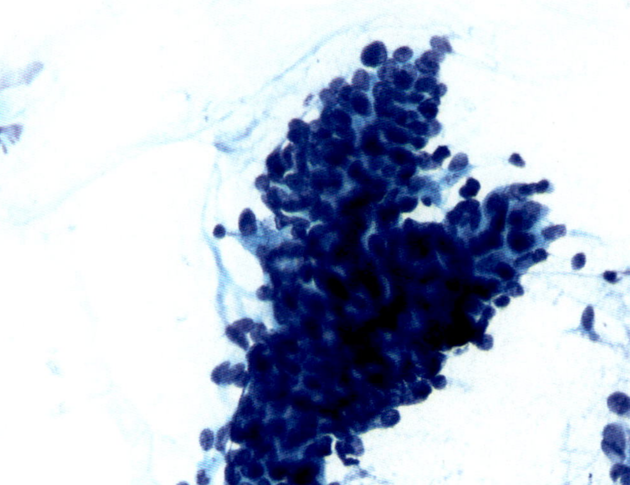

Fig. 9.16. Endometrioid adenocarcinoma showing atypical vacuoles. Pap, 60×.

Fig. 9.18. Liquid-based preparation of endometrial adenocarcinoma. Pap, 40×.

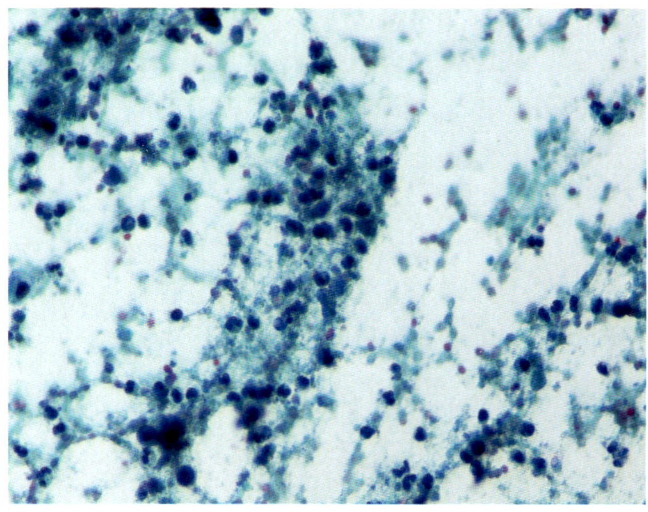

Fig. 9.17. Necrotic debris in endometrial adenocarcinoma. Pap, 40×.

Special care must be exercised in patients with stenosis of the endocervical canal in whom an endometrial biopsy may be difficult or impossible to obtain as an office procedure.

Liquid-Based Preparation
Cancer cells derived from EA should look essentially identical to their counterparts in a conventional smear with the following few differences (fig. 9.18):
– Lack of obvious 'watery diathesis'.
– Three-dimensional arrangements may be accentuated making visualization of the cells within the group difficult.

– Vacuolated or granular cytoplasm.
– Stromal histiocytes and oxyphilic cells.

9.6. Special Types of Malignant Endometrial Epithelial Tumors

The histopathological and cytological features of the different types of EA according to the 2003 WHO histological classification are presented in this section.

9.6.1. Variants of EnA
Several subtypes of EnA occur including squamous, secretory, ciliated and villoglandular variants (table 9.1).

Variant with Squamous Differentiation
Concept. Variable amounts of neoplastic epithelium showing squamous differentiation can be identified in 20–50% of EnA.

Histopathology. The commonest pattern of squamous differentiation in EnA is morules or infiltrating nests similar to conventional squamous cell carcinoma (fig. 9.19). These tumors were formerly classified as adenoacanthoma and adenosquamous carcinoma respectively, but these terms are no longer used. The behavior of EnA with squamous differentiation depends on the type and grade of glandular component and on the depth of myometrial invasion, as in typical EnA.

Cytopathology. Both types of cells can be found in EBT. Malignant glandular cells dominate the smear and may show

Cytopathology of Endometrial
Adenocarcinoma

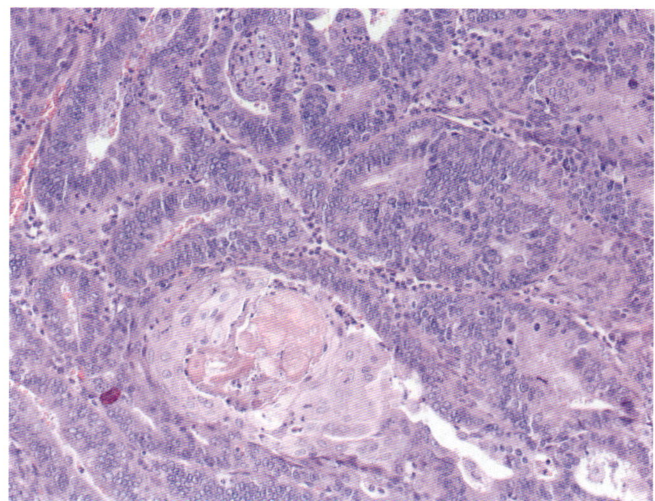
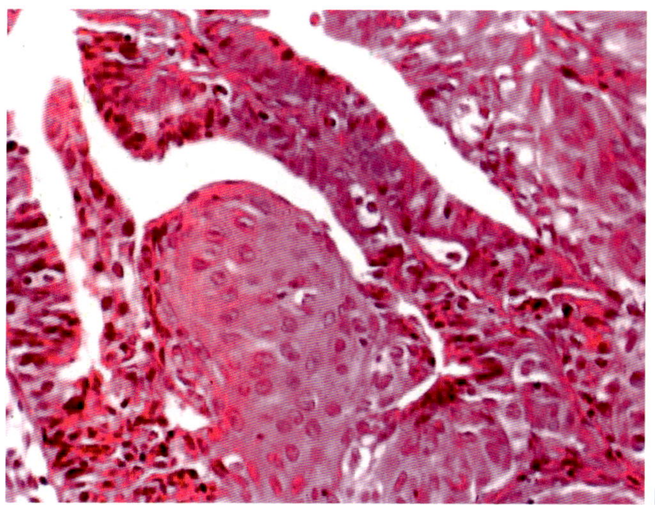

Fig. 9.19. Endometrioid adenocarcinoma with squamous differentiation: **a** Benign squamous component. Histology: HE, 20×. **b** Malignant squamous component. Histology: HE, 40×.

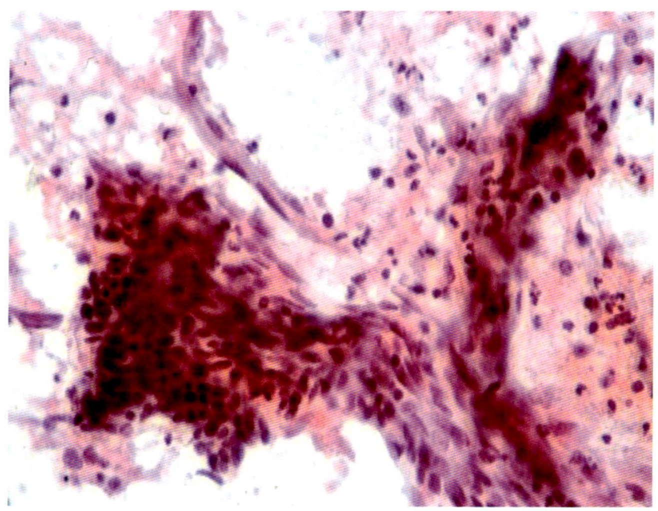

Fig. 9.20. Endometrial brushing of endometrial carcinoma with squamous differentiation. Pap, 40×.

the spectrum from well to poorly-differentiated. Squamous cells forming morules, or metaplastic and malignant squamous epithelial cells usually of the non-keratinizing but also of the keratinizing type can all be found (fig. 9.20). Koss and Melamed [106] noted that the squamous cells usually differ somewhat from cells of cervical carcinoma, the cytoplasm of which is sometimes densely keratinized, called 'keratin bodies'.

Villoglandular Variant
Concept. The villoglandular variant accounts for 13–31% of EnA and usually involves part of a low-grade EnA.

Histopathology. Villoglandular carcinoma is characterized by the usual malignant endometrial cells forming villous fronds with delicate central stromal cores (fig. 9.21). It is not difficult to distinguish from the complex papillary architecture of serous and clear-cell endometrial adenocarcinoma (CCEA). The behavior is similar to that of typical EnA [33, 232].

Cytopathology. Smears from villoglandular EnA are distinguished from smears of other variants by the presence of prominent papillae in many more cellular specimens. The papillary cell clusters are composed of large cells with abundant eosinophilic cytoplasm and large pale nuclei with visible nucleoli. Necrosis in the background is more frequently associated with bare nuclei [225] (fig. 9.21).

9.6.2. Mucinous Adenocarcinoma
Concept. A primary EA, the cells of which contain a significant amount of intracytoplasmic mucin. This is a rare variant, about 1% of all EA [33]. Since it is usually diagnosed in stage I, mucinous adenocarcinoma (MA) has a favorable prognosis similar to other low-grade EA.

Histopathology. MA is the only endometrial tumor that contains intracytoplasmic mucin. According to WHO criteria, >90% of the tumor should be composed of mucin-secreting cells. Mucin-filled glands are also found. The histopathological pattern is similar to primary MA of the endocervix, which is a more common tumor and has to be ruled out before a primary endometrial MA is diagnosed.

Cytopathology. The endometrial smear shows neoplastic endometrial cells with intracytoplasmic mucin seen as vacuoles of varying size. In Pap, the mucin has an eosinophilic

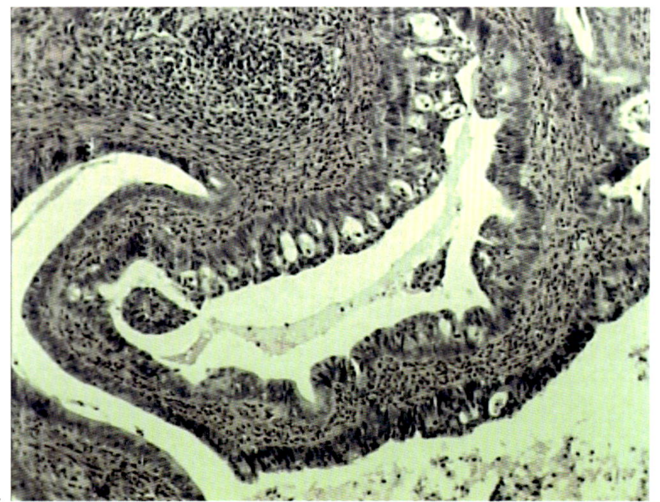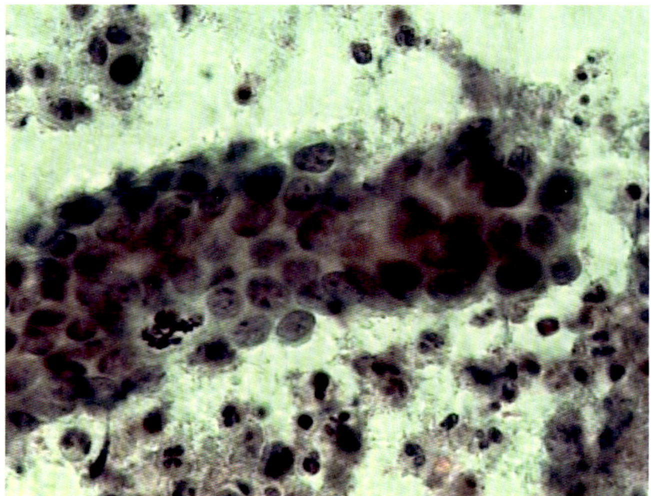

Fig. 9.21. Villoglandular variant of endometrioid adenocarcinoma. **a** Histopathology: HE, 20×, and **b** cytology: Pap, 60×.

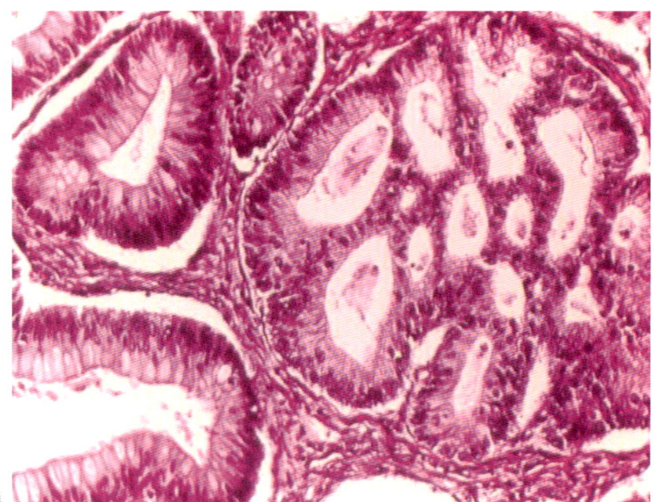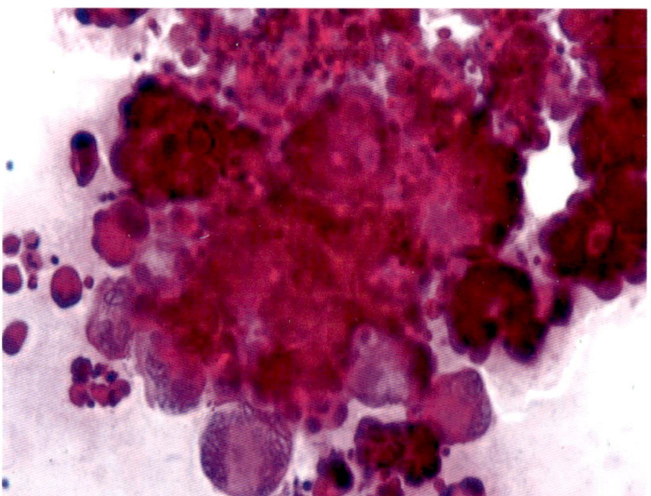

Fig. 9.22. Mucinous endometrial adenocarcinoma. **a** Histopathology: HE, 40×, and **b** cytology: PAS, 40×.

appearance. It can be confirmed by staining with muci-carmine (fig. 9.22). Mucicarmine-positive material can also be found extracellularly and occasionally in signet-ring cells. Less atypical cancer cells appear in papillary clusters with irregular polarity.

9.6.3. Serous Endometrial Adenocarcinoma

Concept. A primary adenocarcinoma of the endometrium with a prominent papillary pattern. Serous endometrial ade-nocarcinoma (SEA) is a high-grade, non-hormone-dependent carcinoma with very aggressive behavior. Grading is not applied to this tumor. It is frequently associated with an

EP [181]. SEA constitutes 5–10% of endometrial cancers and occurs in women 10 years older than women with EnA [33].

Histopathology. SEA has a characteristic papillary pattern with small cellular papillae consisting of fibrovascular stalks covered by stratified epithelial cells and cellular buds. Single cells are often shed from the papillae (fig. 9.23). Psammoma bodies are found in about 30% of patients.

The histopathology of SEA closely resembles that of ovar-ian papillary serous carcinoma including a multicentric pat-tern of spread over the peritoneal surface. This mode of spreading is similar to highly aggressive ovarian surface

Cytopathology of Endometrial
Adenocarcinoma

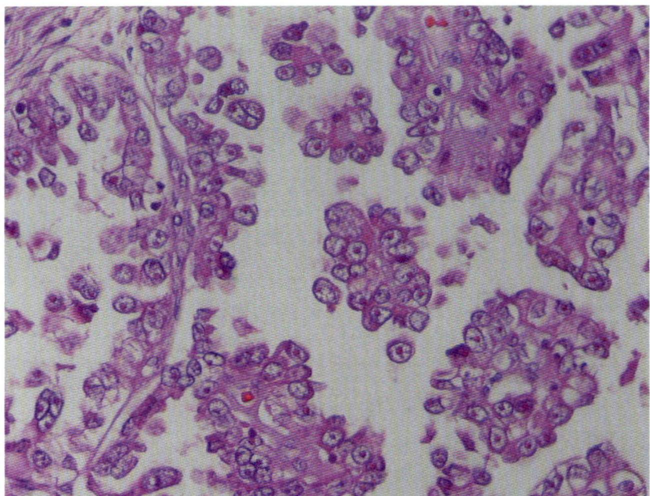

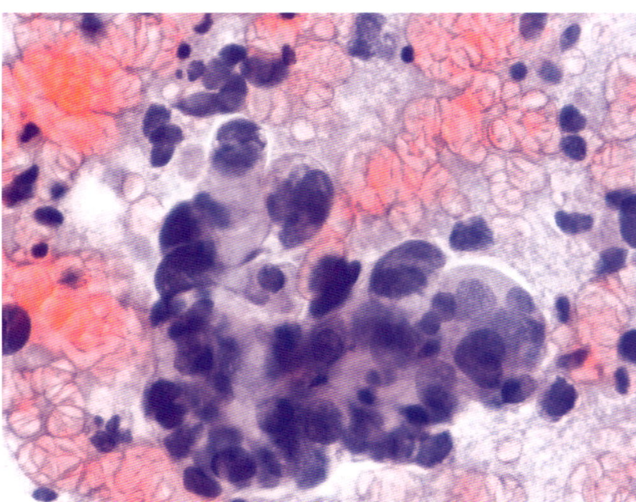

Fig. 9.23. Serous endometrial adenocarcinoma. Histopathology: HE, 40×.

Fig. 9.24. Serous adenocarcinoma. Pap, 60×.

epithelial carcinomas and suggests the need for adjuvant therapy and surgery [78]. Immunohistochemical techniques show an overexpression of the genes p53 and MIB-1.

Cytopathology. CVS of SEA are more likely to contain malignant cells than smears from patients with EnA, due to the papillary architecture and the ease of shedding. Todo et al. [208] found a significantly higher positive rate for smears of SEA: 72.7 vs. 27.4, $p < 0.05$. The predominance of either papillary clusters, bare nuclei or malignant cells is indicative of a possible SEA [225].

A high-grade cytological pattern is obvious in EBT. There is abundant shedding of neoplastic cells in flat sheets, three-dimensional clusters and typical papillae with fibrovascular cores and clustered cells with peripheral moulding. The tumor cells are of two different types. The malignant cells lining the papillae are usually small and show frequent moulding (fig. 9.24). The other type of cell is pleomorphic, showing marked variation in nuclear size, macronucleoli, and sometimes multinucleation. The cytoplasm is dense and well-defined. There is tumoral diathesis with numerous bare nuclei and occasional psammoma bodies in the background.

9.6.4. Clear Cell Endometrial Adenocarcinoma

Concept. CCEA is a malignant tumor composed of clear cells and hobnail cells. It accounts for 1–3% of endometrial carcinomas (EC). It is predominantly seen in postmenopausal women but on rare occasions in young patients [224]. It is included in the EC type II category, and is usually diagnosed at an advanced stage with a poor prognosis. This tumor is also not graded.

Histopathology. CCEA is morphologically, by light and electron microscopy, similar to clear-cell carcinoma anywhere in the female genital tract. The architectural pattern is tubular, papillary, solid or mixed. The clear cells are polygonal and have abundant clear, glycogen-rich cytoplasm and eccentric pleomorphic nuclei. The clear cells and the hobnail cells protrude into lumina and papillary spaces, and are associated with stromal hyalinization (fig. 9.25).

Cytopathology. Smears generally show the pattern of EA. Distinctive features of CCEA are only seen in some cases. In such patients, spherical aggregates of cells arranged in a monolayer form (the so-called 'mirror ball pattern') can be found besides clusters of adenocarcinoma cells of irregular size. The cytoplasm appears translucent and clear or vacuolated (glycogen). Nuclei are large and pleomorphic and may be central or located eccentrically (hobnail nuclei). Both types of nuclei have prominent nucleoli. (fig. 9.25).

9.6.5. Mixed Adenocarcinoma

Mixed EA is defined as a tumor which contains both type I (endometrioid or mucinous carcinoma) and a type II (serous or clear-cell) component. The minor component must involve at least 10% of the total volume of the tumor. A relatively high proportion of the aggressive type II component usually carries a poor prognosis that requires adjuvant therapy.

9.6.6. Primary Squamous Cell Carcinoma of the Endometrium

Concept. A primary carcinoma of the endometrium composed of malignant squamous epithelial cells of varying degrees of differentiation. It is an uncommon tumor, about

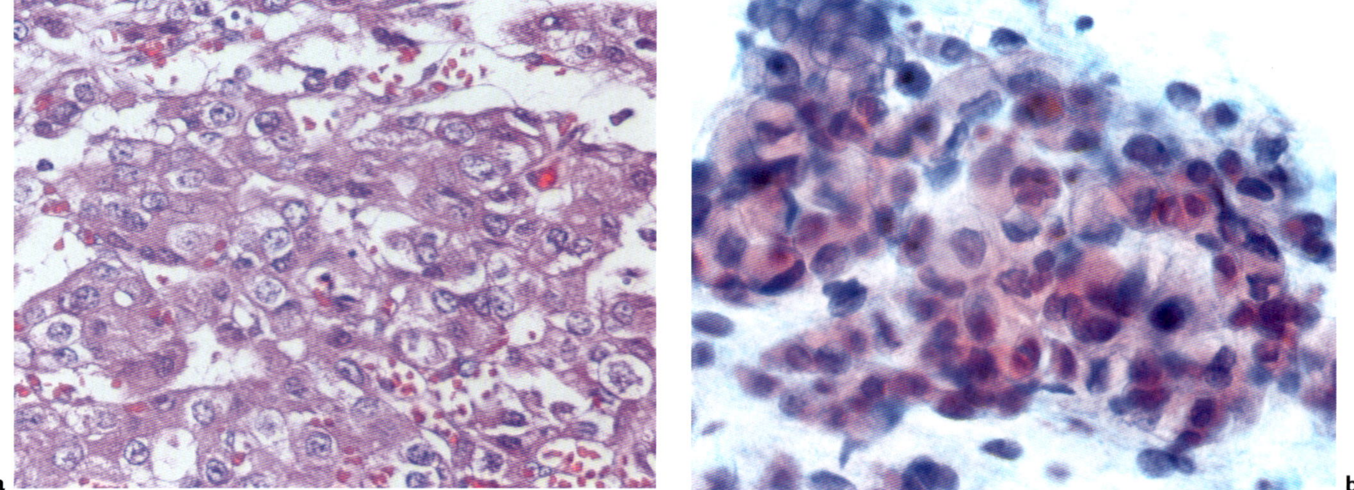

Fig. 9.25. Clear-cell endometrial adenocarcinoma. **a** Histopathology: HE, 40×, and **b** cytology: Pap, 60×.

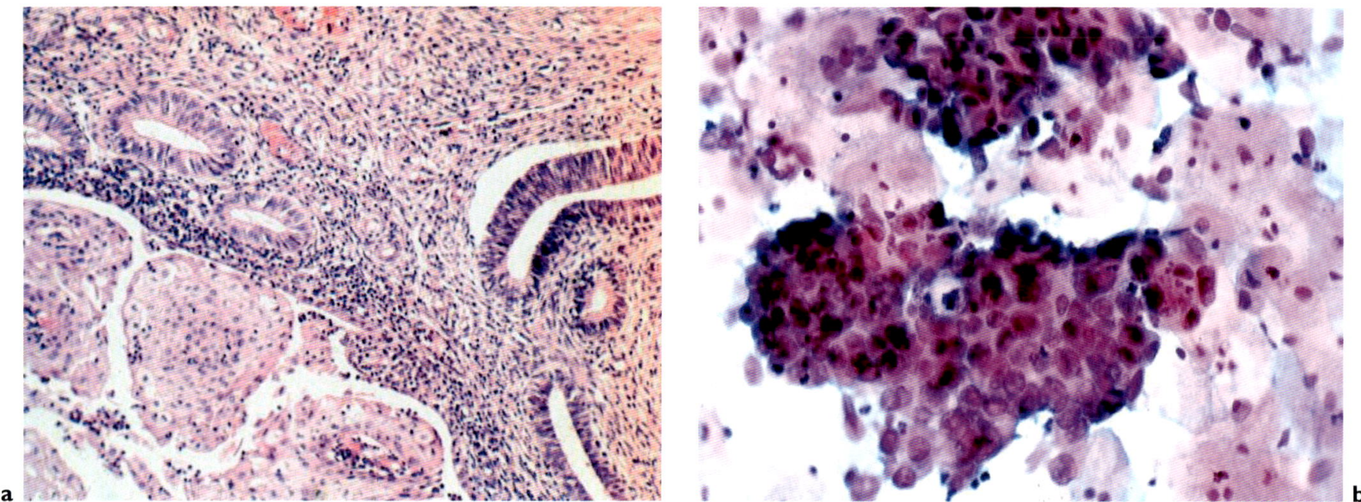

Fig. 9.26. Primary squamous cell carcinoma of the endometrium. **a** Histopathology: HE, 20×, and **b** cytology: Pap, 60×.

0.5% of EC. Almost all of these tumors occur in the post-menopausal age group. Chronic pyometra with cervical stenosis and multiparity seem to be predisposing factors. Data regarding the relationship between HPV status and primary squamous cell carcinoma of the endometrium (PSCCE) are contradictory. HPV has been detected in rare cases of carcinoma [33, 81, 84]. The prognosis of PSCCE is poorer than that of EC and cervical squamous cell carcinoma.

Histopathology. The histopathology is identical to that of cervical squamous cell carcinoma (fig. 9.26) including a rare verrucous variant, which also has a good prognosis in this site [68]. The absence of squamous neoplasia in the exo- and endocervix and of a cervical squamous cell carcinoma extending into the endometrium must be excluded before making a confident diagnosis of PSCCE.

Cytopathology. There are no cytological signs specific for PSCCE and smears could show the same three types of squamous cell carcinoma as seen in the cervix. The source of the cytological sample, and the fact that EC sheds fewer cells, could help in the distinction from cervical squamous cell

Cytopathology of Endometrial
Adenocarcinoma

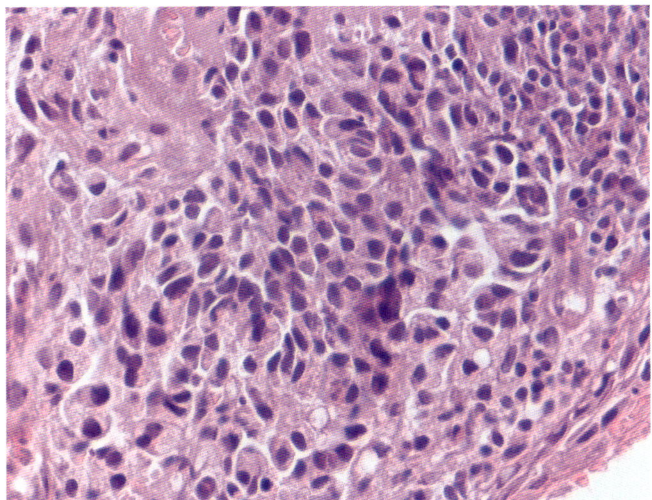

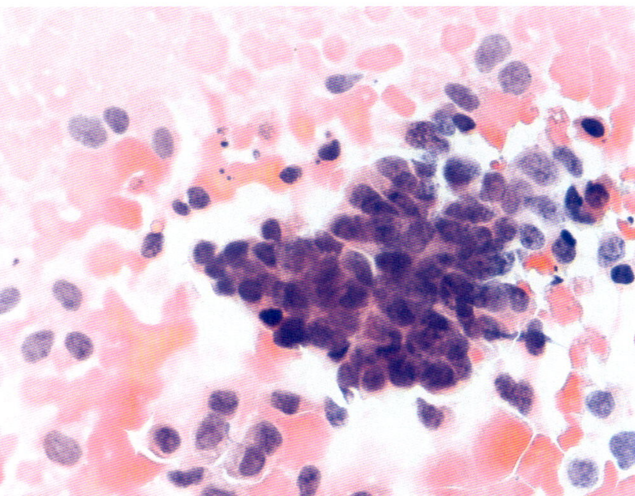

Fig. 9.27. Small cell carcinoma of the endometrium. Histology: HE, 40×>

Fig. 9.28. Small cell carcinoma of the endometrium. Cytology: Pap, 60×.

carcinoma. Although the incidence of abnormal Pap smears in PSCCE is not high, its diagnosis must be considered in any postmenopausal woman whose Pap contains malignant squamous epithelial cells and in whom colposcopy and cervical biopsies are negative [45].

9.6.7. Small Cell Carcinoma

Concept. An EC resembling small cell carcinoma (SmCC) of the lung. It is an uncommon tumor which accounts for <1% of all carcinomas of the endometrium. It has a high propensity for systemic spread and, like its cervical counterpart, has a poor prognosis.

Histopathology. Similar to that of SmCC in other organs, it presents sheets, cords, nests and rosettes of small or intermediate-size cells, with scanty cytoplasm, hyperchromatic nuclei and mitotic figures (fig. 9.27). It is positive for keratin and neuroendocrine markers (WHO [33]) and electron microscopy reveals cytoplasmic neurosecretory granules [209].

Cytopathology. The cytology is identical to that of SmCC of the lung or cervix. In Pap or EBT, tumor cells are small and single or arranged in groups. The cytoplasm is scanty, barely visible, and the dark nuclei show typical moulding, finely stippled chromatin and inconspicuous nucleoli (fig. 9.28). Tumor diathesis is common. If small cell uterine carcinoma is suspected in a CVS, the similarity between cervical and endometrial SmCC necessitates colposcopy, differential curettage and demonstration of neuroendocrine markers [171].

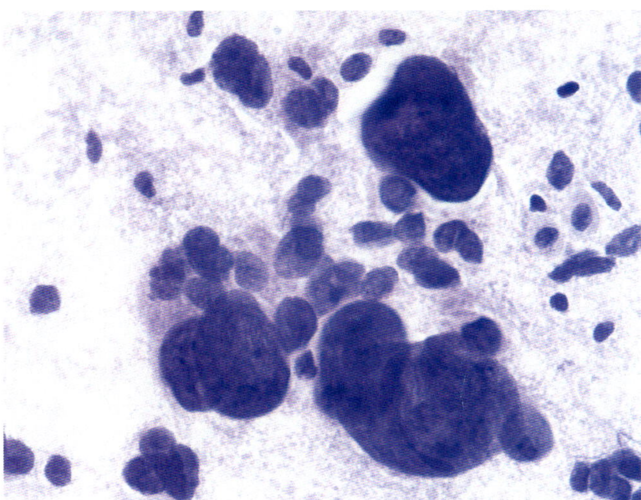

Fig. 9.29. Undifferentiated carcinoma of the endometrium. Pap, 60×.

9.6.8. Undifferentiated Carcinoma

Undifferentiated carcinoma is defined as an EC that is too poorly differentiated to be included in any of the other subtypes (WHO). This category accounts for 1.6–1.8% of EC in the postmenopausal age group. About one half of undifferentiated carcinomas belong to the large-cell type and the rest are indeterminate or small-cell types [33]. The histopathological and cytopathological patterns are in concordance with the types of undifferentiated carcinoma mentioned above (fig. 9.29).

Table 9.6. Differential diagnosis of endometrial adenocarcinoma

Benign processes:
– Endometrial polyp
– Chronic endometritis
– Arias-Stella reaction
– Reactive endocervical cells
– IUD effects
– Microglandular hyperplasia of the cervix
– Effects of hormone therapy

Table 9.7. Differential diagnosis of endometrial adenocarcinoma

Malignant tumors:
1. Epithelial tumors
a. Primary tumors
   – Endocervical adenocarcinoma
   – Extra-uterine adenocarcinoma
   – Squamous cell carcinoma
b. Secondary tumors metastatic from
   – Ovary
   – Fallopian tube
   – Breast
   – Gastrointestinal tract
   – Pancreas

2. Non-epithelial tumors
a. Mesenchymal tumors
   – Leiomyosarcoma
   – Endometrial stromal sarcoma
b. Malignant müllerian mixed tumors
c. Gestational trophoblastic tumors
   – Choriocarcinoma

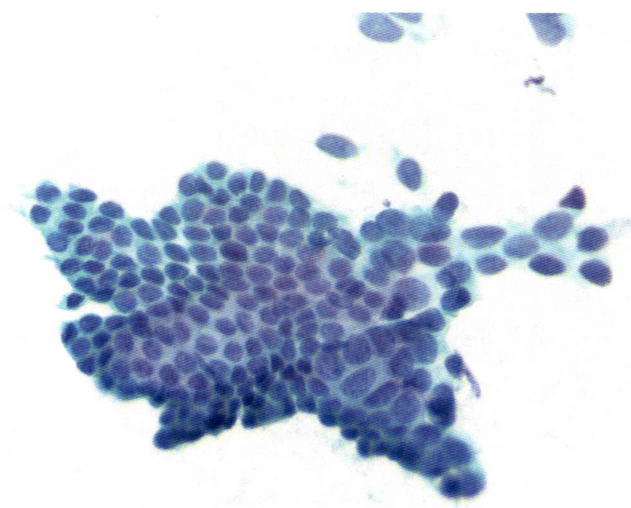

Fig. 9.30. Endometrial polyp. Pap, 60×.

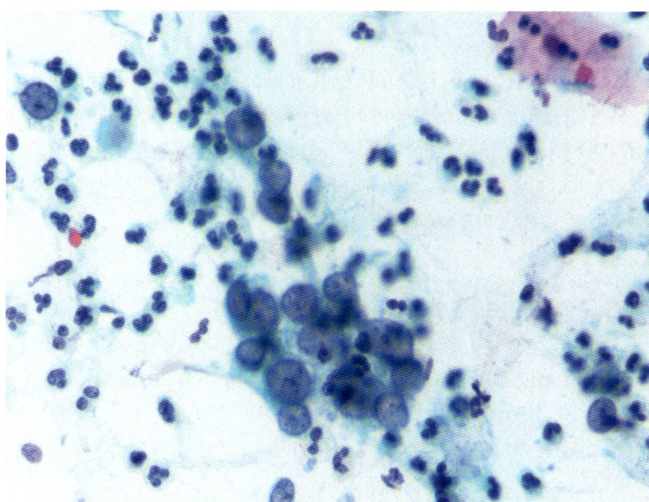

Fig. 9.31. Arias-Stella reaction. Pap, 60×.

9.7. Differential Diagnosis of Endometrial Adenocarcinoma

Tables 9.6 and 9.7 list the most important differential diagnoses of EA in cytological smears. The benign processes to be considered in the differential diagnosis are listed in table 9.6, the malignant tumors in table 9.7. The differential diagnosis between EA and different types of EH has been discussed in Chapter 8.

9.7.1. Benign Processes

9.7.1.1. Endometrial Polyp
Some EP may undergo an atypical ulceration, which in a few cases may exfoliate endometrial sheets with significant atypia (fig. 9.30). This may cause problems in the differential diagnosis between a polyp and EA, both in an EBT and in an endometrial curettage [22, 206].

9.7.1.2. Chronic Endometritis
Chronic non-specific endometritis yields numerous lymphocytes and irregular endometrial cell clusters in EBT (fig. 7.1). The inflammatory process may induce reactive changes in the endometrial cells, including nuclear atypia. The hallmark of chronic non-specific endometritis is the presence of endometrial stromal cells closely admixed with scattered and clustered plasma cells [146, 151]. In tuberculous endometritis, some endometrial epithelial cells may show reactive changes with nuclear irregularity and hyperchromasia

Cytopathology of Endometrial
Adenocarcinoma

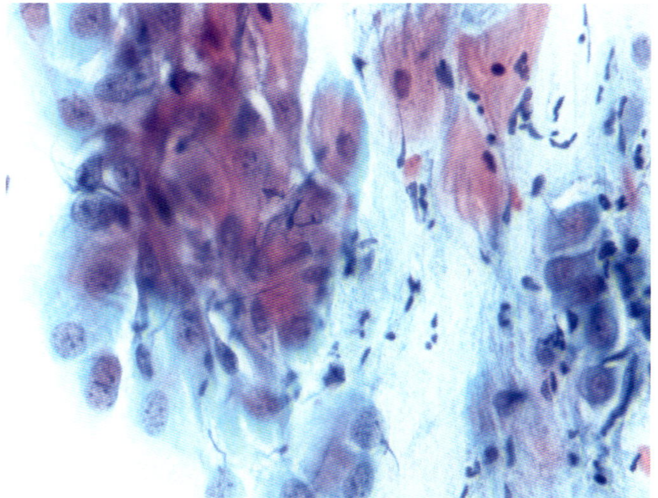

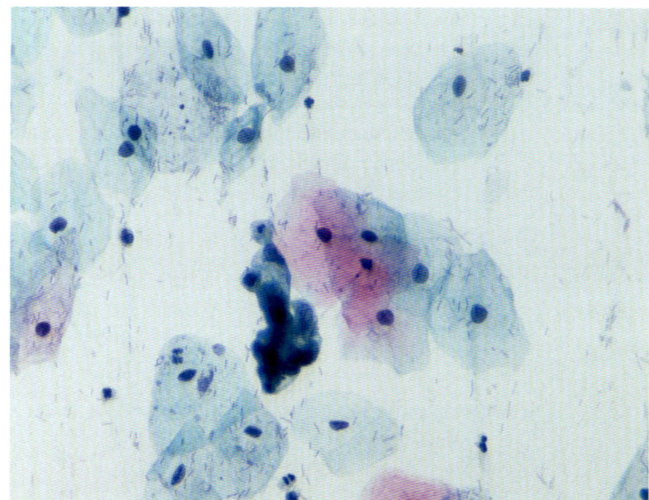

Fig. 9.32. Reactive endocervical cells. Pap, 60×.

Fig. 9.33. IUD effects. Pap, 40×.

mimicking carcinoma cells. Multinucleated Langhans' giant cells help in the diagnosis of tuberculosis. The inflammatory effect could be associated with some changes in endometrial cells such as cytoplasmic vacuolation and nuclear hyperchromasia, resembling regenerative endometrium post curettage.

9.7.1.3. Arias-Stella Reaction

An Arias-Stella reaction of glandular epithelium can on rare occasions be found in a CVS, mostly in relation to pregnancy. The glandular cells have enlarged, hyperchromatic and eccentrically located nuclei with macronucleoli and vacuolated cytoplasm mimicking adenocarcinoma cells, especially of the clear-cell type (fig. 9.31). The absence of overlapping and stratification of the cells points to the diagnosis of an Arias-Stella reaction rather than CCEA. As a practical conclusion, these benign changes have to be considered before diagnosing carcinoma in a young pregnant patient [50].

9.7.1.4. Reactive Endocervical Cells

Reactive endocervical cells including atypical repair can look like CA or EA but show more marked variation of nuclear and nucleolar size and shape than these tumors. In favor of reparative cells is the absence of individual cells with suspicious features. In addition, reparative cells are larger, and have a dense cytoplasm and a thin nuclear membrane in contrast to the thick and irregular nuclear membranes seen in EA (fig. 9.32). The reactive cells occur in sheets but do not form cell balls typical of EA [31].

9.7.1.5. IUD Effects

Pap from some users of IUD may contain glandular cells with features morphologically indistinguishable from those

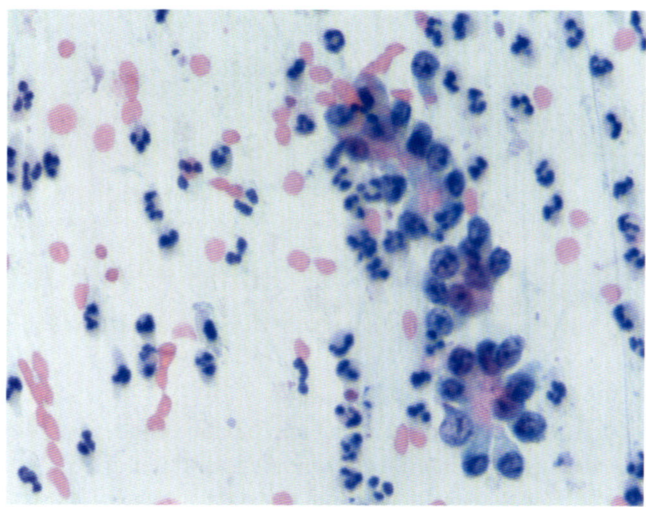

Fig. 9.34. Microglandular hyperplasia of the cervix. Pap, 60×.

of EA (fig. 9.33). It is important that the cytology laboratory is informed if the patient has an IUD.

9.7.1.6. Microglandular Hyperplasia of the Cervix

This benign proliferation of the endocervical glands has points in common with the Arias-Stella reaction but not with clear cell carcinoma. Pregnancy and oral contraceptive use may produce marked cytological atypia. This could lead to the diagnosis of AGC and may resemble the cytological pattern of adenocarcinoma, adenocarcinoma in situ and CA, and also of EA. Cytoplasmic vacuolation with phagocytosed neutrophils and macronucleoli are cytological signs common to EA and microglandular hyperplasia (fig. 9.34). The presence

Table 9.8. Uterine adenocarcinoma

Cytological features	Endocervical	Endometrial
Microarchitecture	Palisading cells	Acini, small clusters, single cells
Shape of cells	Columnar	Cuboidal, rounded
Cell size	Larger than endometrial	Smaller
Cytoplasm	Eosinophilic, granular	Cyanophilic, vacuolated
Nuclear size	10–12 μm	8–10 μm
Nuclear chromatin	Coarse	Finely granular
Nucleoli	Macronucleoli common	Macronucleoli rare

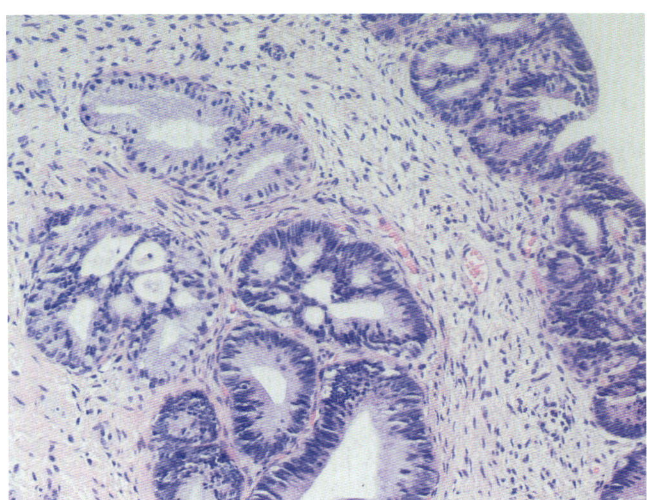 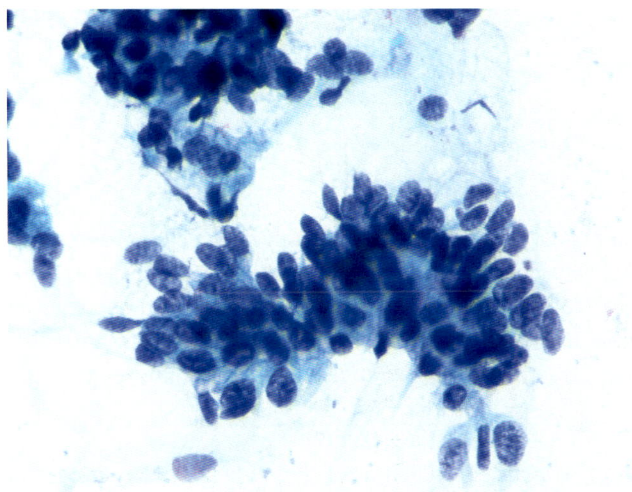

Fig. 9.35. Endocervical adenocarcinoma in situ. **a** Histology; HE, 20×, and **b** cytology: Pap, 60×.

of typical cell clusters showing microlumina and fenestrated spaces was first described by Alvarez-Santín et al. [3] as a specific cytologic pattern of microglandular hyperplasia.

9.7.1.7. Effects of Hormonal Therapy

Single endocervical cells with enlarged hyperchromatic nuclei may appear in women receiving contraceptive hormones with a high progestin content, making a differential diagnosis difficult. EBT or curettage should be recommended in this situation. The clinician should inform the cytology laboratory of the type of hormonal therapy the patient receives.

9.7.2. *Malignant Tumors* (table 9.7)

9.7.2.1. Epithelial Tumors

Endocervical Adenocarcinoma (CA). Among the malignant epithelial tumors, the distinction between EA and CA is the main differential diagnostic problem. Table 9.8 shows the cytological features seen in Pap, which indicate if the adenocarcinoma is located in the endometrium or in the endocervix (fig. 9.35) [99]. However, it is commonly agreed that this may be impossible to decide in some cases. Such cases can be reported as uterine adenocarcinoma with a comment on the most likely location. A D&C is a practical way to solve the problem [31, 150]. The detection of HPV in a Pap and in D&C favors endocervical origin, but it has only been found in between 45 and 70% of the CA [82]. Bonfiglio and Clary [19] reported that the usual types of CA (mucinous) are high-risk HPV-positive in 9% of cases. A panel of immune markers including vimentin, ER/PR and CEA is helpful in distinguishing CA and EA [33, 228].

Extrauterine Adenocarcinoma. When adenocarcinoma cells are observed in a CVS, an extrauterine primary adenocarcinoma should be considered if the following features are present:

– Scant papillary clusters of tumor cells with larger nuclei and less vacuolated cytoplasm than those typical of EA (fig. 9.36) [96].

Cytopathology of Endometrial
Adenocarcinoma

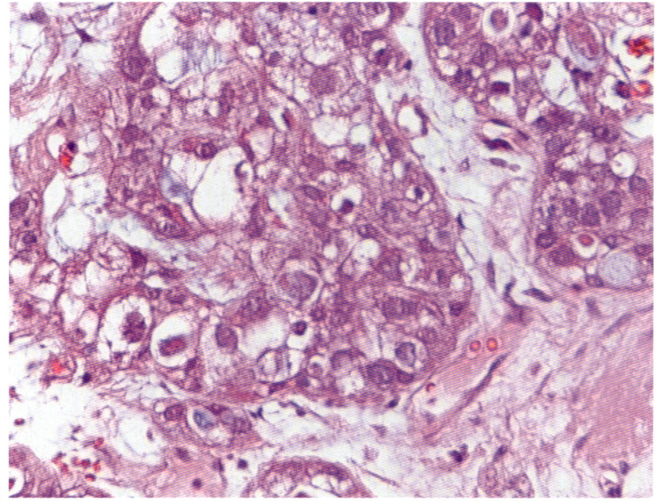

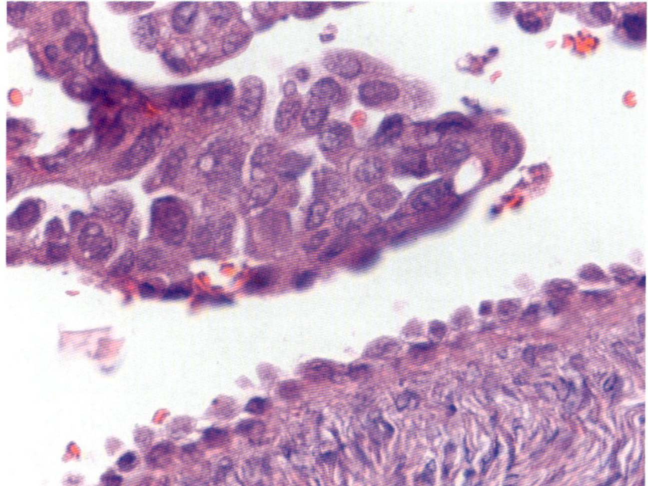

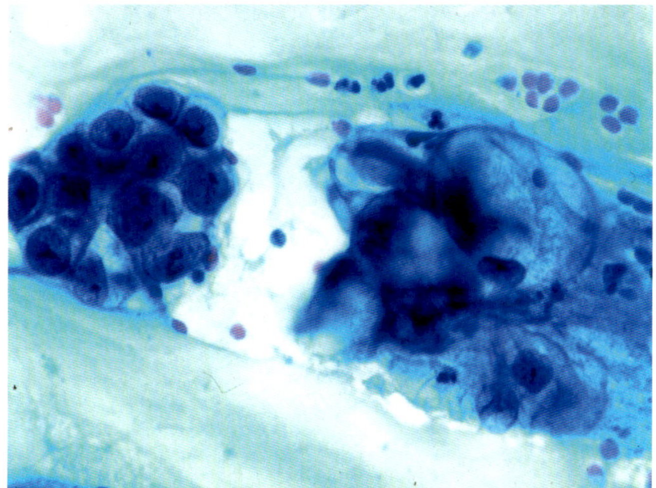

Fig. 9.36. Extrauterine adenocarcinoma. Metastasis of seropapillary adenocarcinoma of the ovary on the surface of an endocervical polyp. **a** Histology polyp: HE, 40×; **b** histology ovary: 40×, and **c** cytology: Pap, 60×.

– Benign findings in cytological and histological specimens from the endometrium.
– The importance of the presence of tumor diathesis is subject to debate [73, 97].
– In most cases of extrauterine adenocarcinoma, the primary site is in the ovary (fig. 9.36) or rarely in the fallopian tube (Jiménez-Ayala) [71].

Squamous Cell Carcinoma. Some well-differentiated EA can mimic cervical carcinoma in situ. The presence of nucleoli and/or tumoral diathesis excludes the diagnosis of cervical carcinoma in situ. A large cell non-keratinizing squamous cell carcinoma should be considered in the differential diagnosis if there are isolated malignant cells or if the cells are arranged in syncytial groups. Cells forming papillary clusters or balls as in EA are not seen in squamous cell carcinoma or in SmCC of the cervix (fig. 9.37).

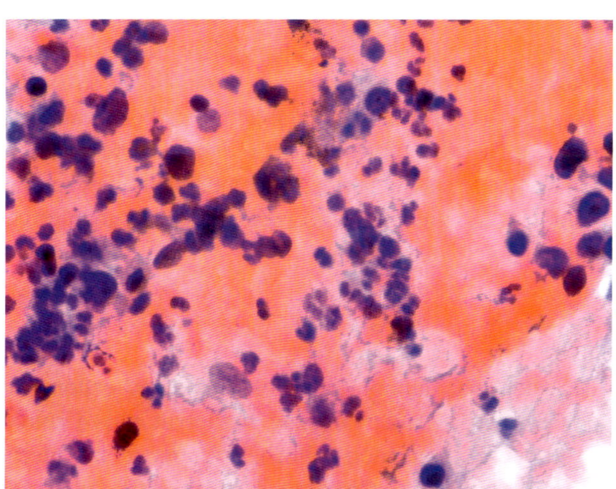

Fig. 9.37. Small cell carcinoma of the cervix. Pap, 60×.

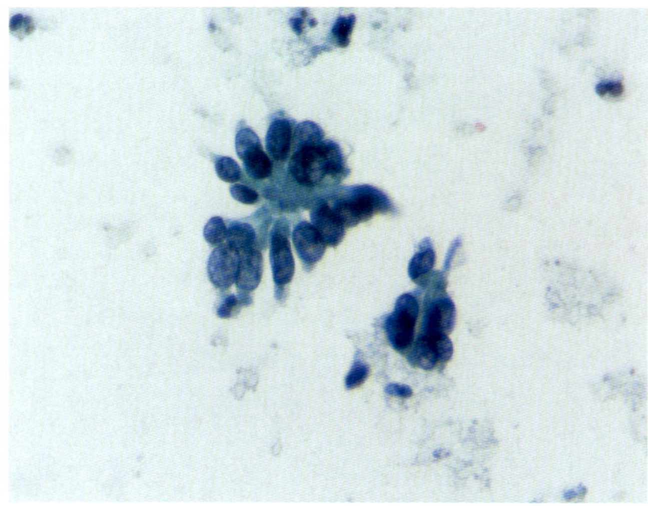

Fig. 9.38. Secondary tumors. Vaginal metastasis of adenocarcinoma of the colon. Pap, 40×.

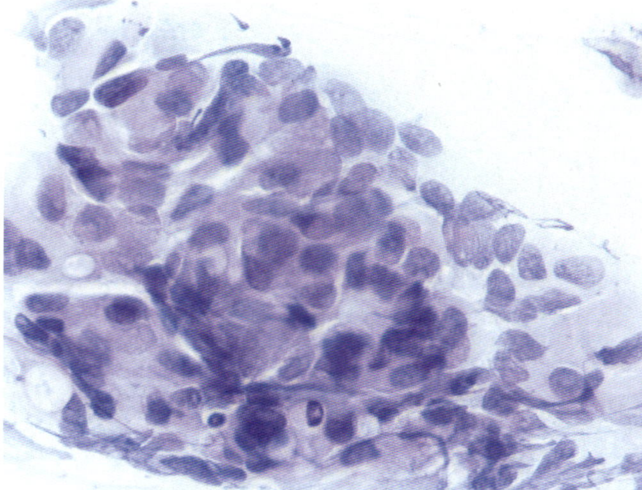

Fig. 9.39. Mesenchymal tumor. Endometrial stromal sarcoma. Pap, 60×.

Secondary Epithelial Tumors. In tumors metastatic to the uterus, malignant cells found in CVS and EBT are mostly of glandular type. The possibility of metastatic tumor should be considered if the malignant cells are associated with some of the following features:
- Tumor diathesis absent.
- The type of tumor cells differs from those seen in the genital tract. The cells may shed as spherical clusters or papillary structures.
- Ascites present.
- A history of cancer of a neighboring organ.

Tumors of the gastrointestinal tract are the most common source of metastasis to the endometrium (fig. 9.38), followed in frequency by breast, skin (melanoma) and lung. The presence of signet-ring cells is more suggestive of gastric carcinoma than of primary EnA. Papillary structures point to the ovary, although mesothelioma and papillary carcinoma of the thyroid or pancreas can also produce similar structures. Some authors [31] point out that psammoma bodies are commonly found in secondary adenocarcinoma of the ovary and fallopian tube. In our experience, psammoma bodies are only very rarely found in Pap and if present they are not always a feature of a malignant tumor.

9.7.2.2. Mesenchymal Tumors and Carcinosarcoma (table 9.7)

Mesenchymal tumors (leiomyosarcoma and endometrial stromal sarcoma) and malignant müllerian mixed tumors (carcinosarcoma) are non-epithelial tumors of the uterine body and should be differentiated from EA in cytological smears. Malignant cells from the first group of tumors occur

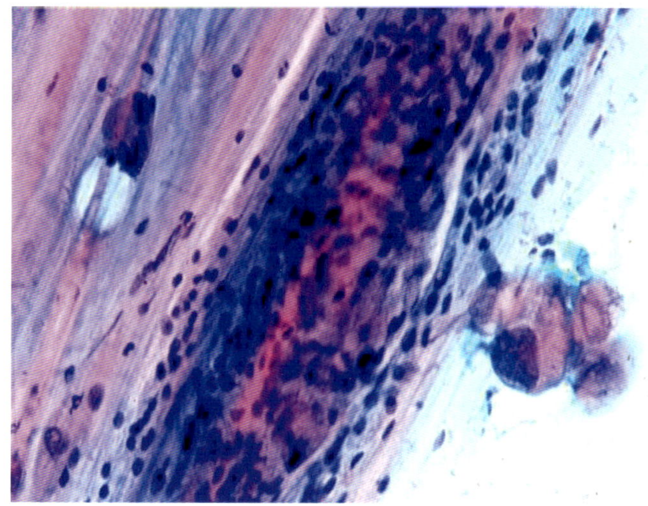

Fig. 9.40. Choriocarcinoma. Endometrial cytology: Pap, 60×.

sparsely, isolated or in small sheets (fig. 9.39), contrary to the mainly larger groups and papillary clusters of EA. Frequently the nuclei are polylobated or multiple and have prominent macronucleoli.

9.7.2.3. Choriocarcinomas

These malignant gestational tumors are usually associated with a pregnancy. The presence of malignant cells with a morphology similar to that of cytotrophoblastic or syncytiotrophoblastic cells points to the possible diagnosis of choriocarcinoma (fig. 9.40).

Cytopathology of Endometrial
Adenocarcinoma

Chapter 10

Cytopathology of the Non-Epithelial Malignant Tumors of the Uterine Corpus

10.1. Histological Classification of Tumors of the Uterine Corpus (WHO 2003, table 10.1)

The seven different types of tumors of the uterine corpus included in the 2003 WHO Classification are listed in table 10.1. The cytopathology of endometrial adenocarcinoma (EA) has been discussed in Chapter 9, that of endometrial hyperplasia (EH) in Chapter 8, of endometrial polyp (EP) in Chapter 7, and of tamoxifen-related lesions in Chapter 1. We have also commented on the differential diagnosis of epithelial and non-epithelial malignant tumors, malignant gestational trophoblastic disease, mainly choriocarcinoma, and on secondary tumors that may involve the endometrium (Chapter 9). This chapter is devoted to the cytopathology of malignant mixed epithelial and mesenchymal tumors (MMMT), completing the presentation of malignant tumors of the uterine corpus.

10.2. Problems in Cytological Diagnosis

A number of features differ between non-epithelial malignant tumors and endometrial carcinoma (EC):

– *Low incidence:* Only 1.46–6.23%, average about 3%, of malignant uterine tumors fall in this category. The ratio of uterine sarcoma to EC is 1:10–50 [115, 190]. The non-epithelial malignant tumors always affect the endometrium. Some arise in this mucosa, others extend from the myometrium into the endometrium [115].

– It is easy to recognize the malignant cytological features of these tumors but it is usually difficult to identify the cell type.

– Occasional shedding found in the cervicovaginal smears:
  Endometrial stromal sarcoma and leiomyosarcoma.
  Large growth into the endometrial cavity.
  Areas of necrosis.
Malignant Mixed epithelial and mesenchymal tumors.

Polypoid growth.
Sparse shedding.
– Endometrial brushing (EBT) produces the best cytological results.

10.3. Cytological Features of Non-Epithelial Malignant Uterine Tumors

The main cytological features are as follows:

Shedding
Usually only sparse, but tumors with extensive growth and necrosis extending into the uterine cavity show more desquamation, shedding cells that appear in endometrial samples.

The cells are isolated or arranged in small groups in contrast to the cells of EA that form larger groups and papillary aggregates (figs 10.1, 10.2).

Table 10.1. Histological classification of tumors of the uterine corpus (WHO, 2003)

Epithelial tumors and related lesions:
– Endometrial carcinoma
– Endometrial hyperplasia
– Endometrial polyp
– Tamoxifen-related lesions
Mesenchymal tumors
Mixed epithelial and mesenchymal tumors
Gestational trophoblastic disease
Miscellaneous tumors
Lymphoid and hematopoietic tumors
Secondary tumors

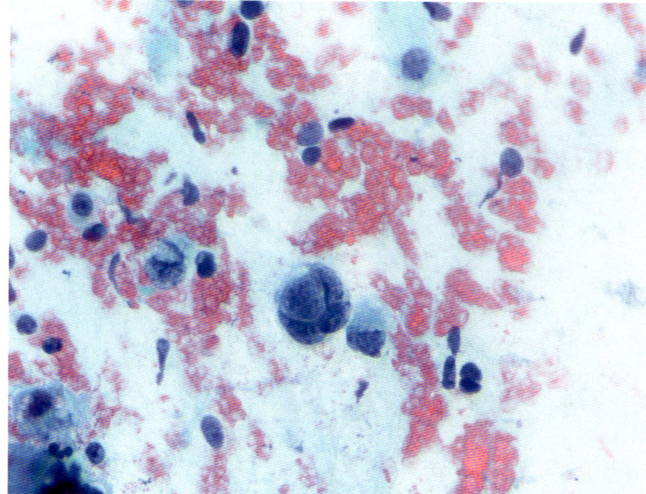

Fig. 10.1. Cytopathology of non-epithelial malignant tumors. Isolated cells in a MMMT. Pap, 60×.

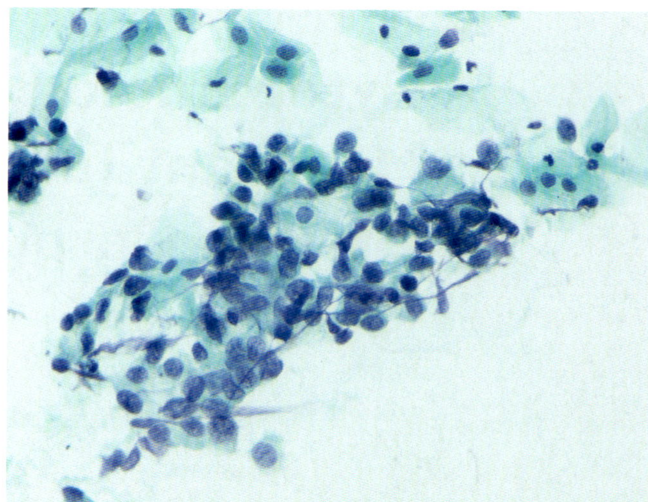

Fig. 10.3. Non-epithelial malignant tumor: group of epithelial cells and mesenchymal cells with bizarre nuclei. Pap, 40×.

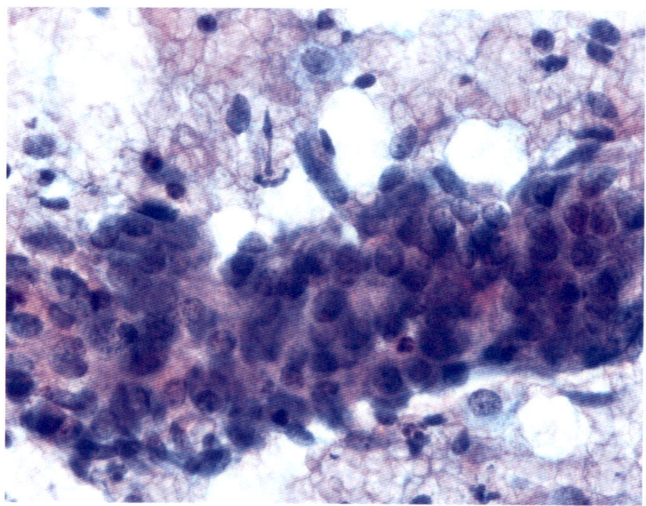

Fig. 10.2. Large aggregate of cells of endometrial adenocarcinoma. Pap, 40×.

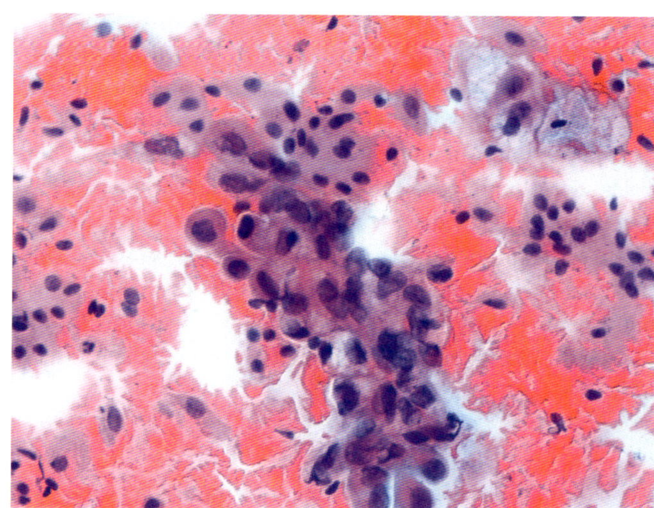

Fig. 10.4. Non-epithelial malignant tumor: anisonucleosis and hyperchromasia. Pap, 40×.

MMMT sheds both malignant epithelial and malignant mesenchymal cells (fig. 10.3).

Nuclei

Chromatin. Nuclear chromatin pattern is variable, finely or coarsely granular, sometimes showing chromatin clumping (fig. 10.4).

Shape and Number. Multilobated nuclei are frequent and multinucleated cells are more frequent than in adenocarcinoma.

Nucleoli. The presence of macronucleoli is one of the most characteristic features of this category of tumors.

Cytoplasm

Size and Shape. Sarcoma cells have abundant cytoplasm and irregular shapes; polygonal, caudate, pleomorphic or fibroblast-like spindle shapes (fig. 10.5).

Structure. The malignant cells exhibit a dense cyanophilic cytoplasm, sometimes with a fibrillar morphology.

Background. Smears show a variable amount of tumoral diathesis (figs 10.6, 10.7). The diathesis is often scanty in mesenchymal malignant tumors (MMT).

Cytopathology of the Non-Epithelial
Malignant Tumors of the Uterine Corpus

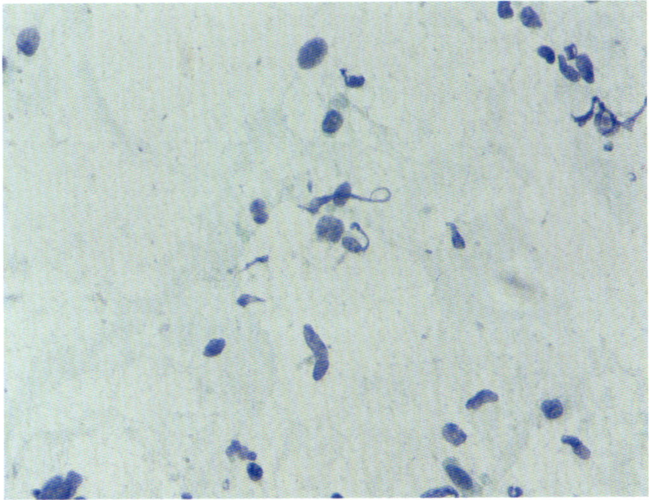

Fig. 10.5. Non-epithelial malignant tumor: spindle cells. Pap, 60×.

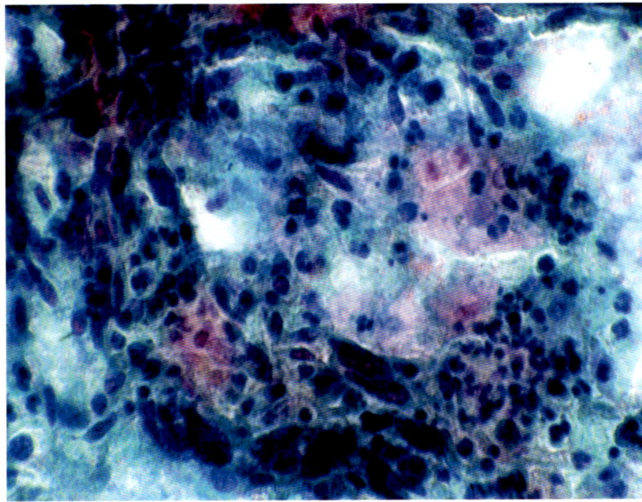

Fig. 10.7. Non-epithelial malignant tumor (leiomyosarcoma): major tumoral diathesis. Pap, 40×.

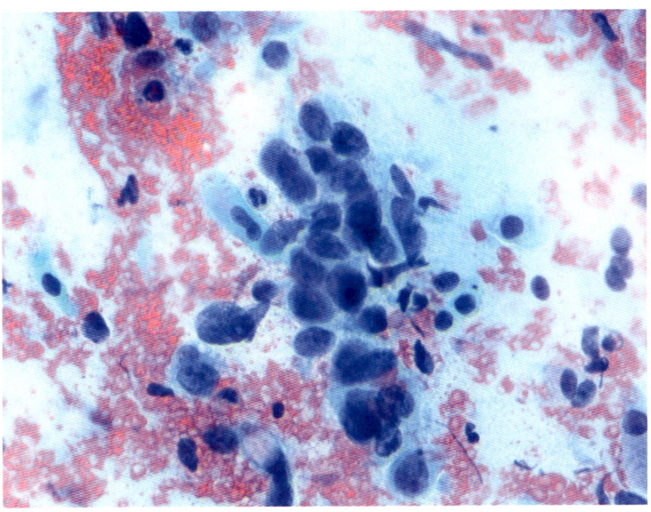

Fig. 10.6. Scanty tumoral diathesis in a non-epithelial malignant tumor. Pap, 40×.

10.4. Mesenchymal Malignant Tumors

MMT constitute about 3% of all malignancies of the uterine corpus. A history of hyperestrogenism and the clinical triad of obesity, hypertension and diabetes seem to be less significant than in EA [204].

There are two types of MMT, endometrial stromal sarcoma (ESS) and leiomyosarcoma (LMS).

Endometrial Stromal Sarcomas

Concept. ESS is a tumor composed of cells that resemble proliferative phase endometrial stromal cells. The WHO 2003 Histological Classification distinguishes two types of ESS: low-grade ESS and undifferentiated endometrial sarcoma (UES). The second type was formerly named high-grade ESS, but this term has been abandoned due to the lack of specific differentiation and because the tumor does not histologically resemble endometrial stroma. The distinction between low-grade ESS and UES is not related to mitotic counts but to nuclear pleomorphism and the presence of necrosis [79].

Clinical Features. ESS occurs in middle-aged women, rarely in younger women. There is no association with risk factors for EA. A few patients have a history of pelvic radiation. Clinical signs are vaginal bleeding and progressively increasing menometrorrhagia [115].

Low-grade ESS is a rare, clinically indolent neoplasm, which constitutes only about 0.2% of all malignant tumors of female genital tract. Its clinical behavior is usually slow growth and late recurrences. UES are aggressive tumors and disseminate rapidly.

Histopathology. Low-grade ESS is a highly cellular tumor of endometrial stroma-type cells showing minimal atypia and a few mitotic figures, and has a plexiform vasculature (figs 10.8, 10.9). UES shows marked cytological atypia and frequent atypical mitotic figures [79] (fig. 10.10).

Cytopathology. ESS is often difficult to diagnose in cytological smears because these tumors usually only shed cells when there is focal tumor necrosis. In UES the problem is in the correct typing of the tumor, which can be mistaken for poorly-differentiated carcinoma and LMS. The distinction between neoplastic cells and benign stromal cells can be a problem in low-grade ESS.

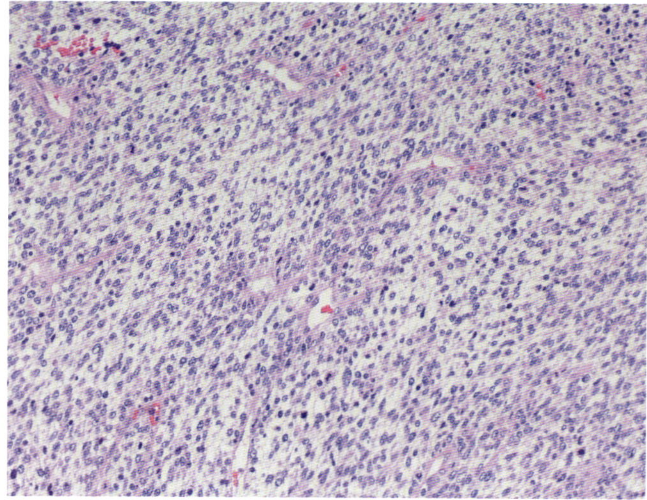

Fig. 10.8. Endometrial stromal sarcoma. Histopathology of a low-grade type. HE, 10×.

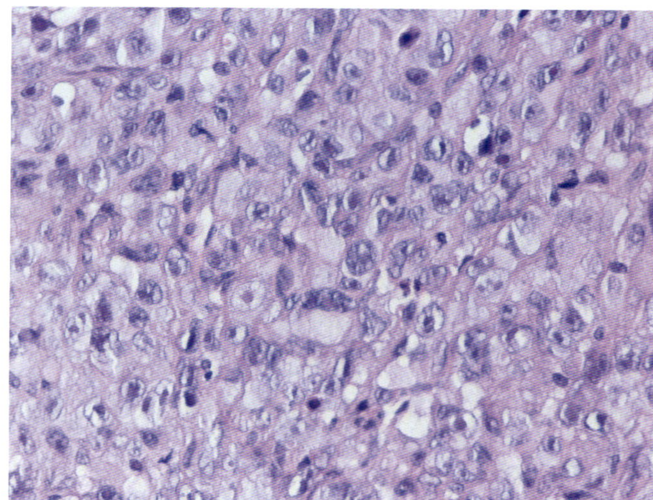

Fig. 10.10. Undifferentiated endometrial sarcoma. Histopathology: HE, 40×.

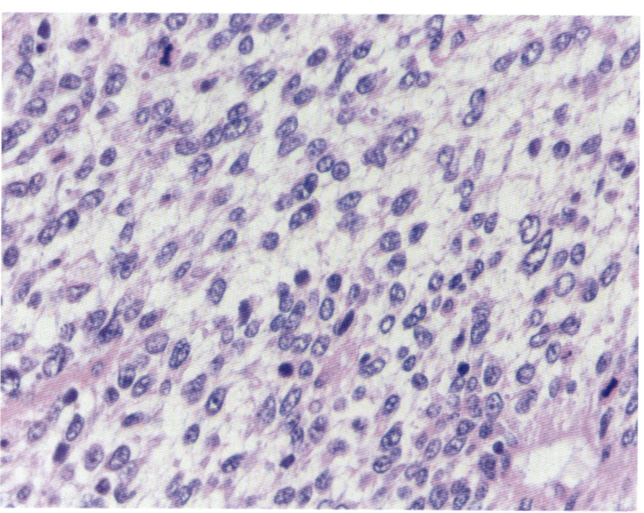

Fig. 10.9. Histopathology of a low-grade ESS. HE, 40×.

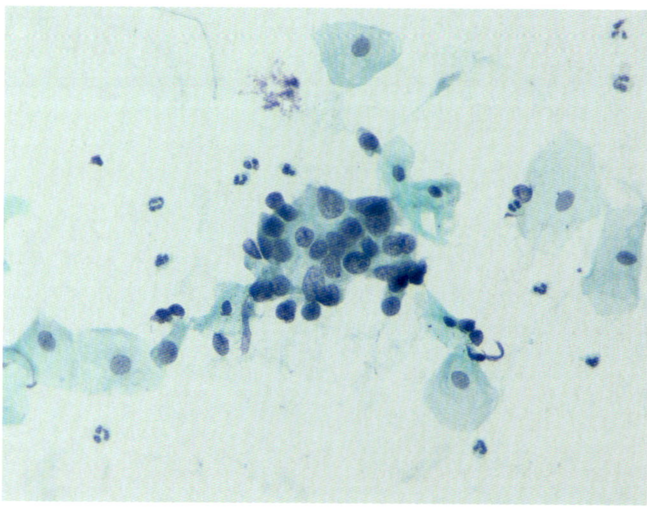

Fig. 10.11. Endometrial stromal sarcoma. Endometrial brushing of a low-grade type. Pap, 40×.

Low-Grade ESS. An abundance of single stromal cells with enlarged nuclei and the absence of glandular cells in an EBT smear are important features that suggest a diagnosis of low-grade ESS [86]. EBT shows neoplastic cells, usually single or in small groups. The cells are small and uniform but show anisokaryosis. Nuclear chromatin is slightly coarse and nucleoli are inconspicuous (fig. 10.11).

UES. The neoplastic cells are usually single or in small groups. There may be bizarre pleomorphic cells with 'comet' forms, spindle cells and giant cells. Nuclei are enlarged with coarsely clumped chromatin and macronucleoli but rarely multinucleated (figs 10.12, 10.13). Mitotic figures are usually found in UES but not in low-grade ESS. The cytoplasm is ill-defined and stripped nuclei are frequent. The smear background shows evident tumor diathesis with debris and phagocytosis (foreign body giant cells).

Differential Diagnosis (table 10.2)

Malignant Tumors

Epithelial Tumors. ESS must be differentiated from the more common epithelial malignant tumors, EA and small cell carcinoma of the cervix (figs 10.14, 10.15). The microarchitectural pattern, the number and distribution of cells, and

Cytopathology of the Non-Epithelial
Malignant Tumors of the Uterine Corpus

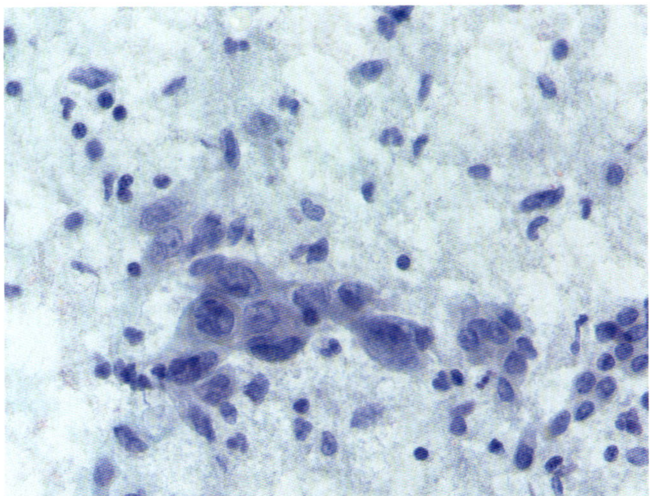

Fig. 10.12. Cytology of undifferentiated endometrial sarcoma. Pap, 60×.

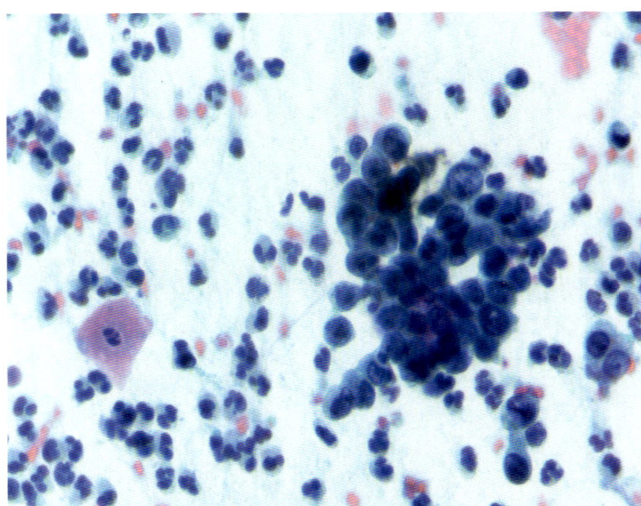

Fig. 10.14. Endometrial adenocarcinoma. Pap, 60×.

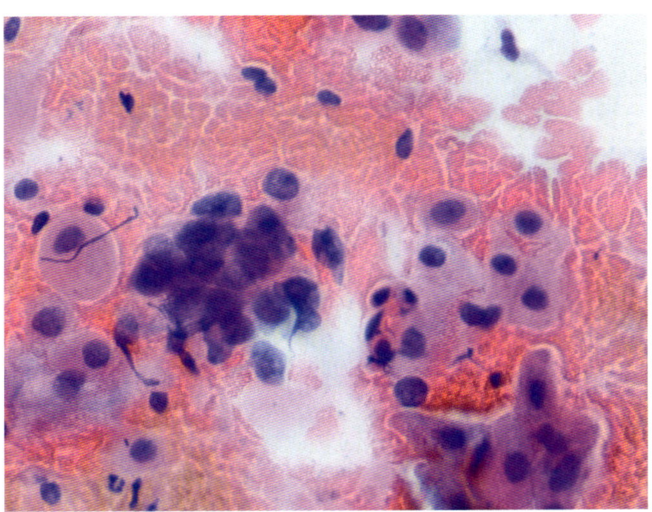

Fig. 10.13. Bizarre cells of an undifferentiated endometrial sarcoma. Pap, 60×.

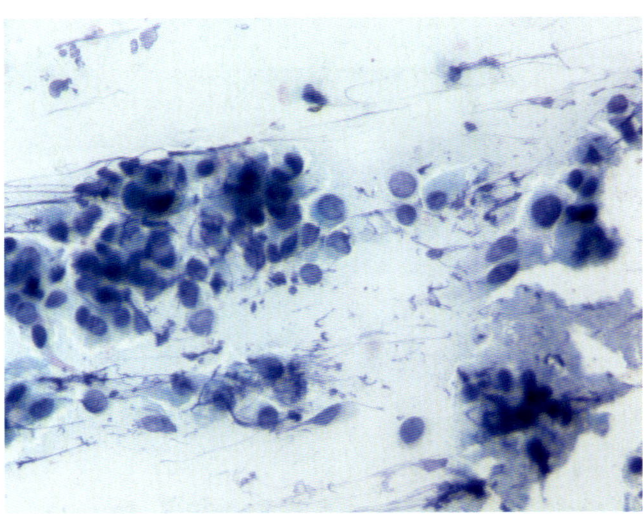

Fig. 10.15. Small cell carcinoma of the cervix. Pap, 60×.

Table 10.2. Endometrial stromal sarcoma. Cytological differential diagnosis

Malignant tumors
- Epithelial tumors:
    Endometrial adenocarcinoma
    Small cell carcinoma of cervix
- Lymphoid tumors:
    Non-Hodgkin lymphoma
- Kaposis sarcoma

Benign lesions
- Follicular cervicitis
- Stromal endometriosis of cervix

the nuclear and cytoplasmic features are all helpful in the differential diagnosis.

Lymphoid Tumors. Malignant cells of non-Hodgkin's lymphoma involving the uterus are monomorphic and mainly dispersed and single, and show little cytoplasm and marked hyperchromasia (fig. 10.16). The expression of leukocyte common antigen is an important clue to the diagnosis.

Kaposi's Sarcoma. The neoplastic cells in Kaposi's sarcoma are spindle-shaped resembling fibroblast. They show a high mitotic activity and variable nuclear atypia. ESS is associated with profuse vaginal bleeding and an enlarged uterus on pelvic examination. ESS usually exhibits deep endometrial

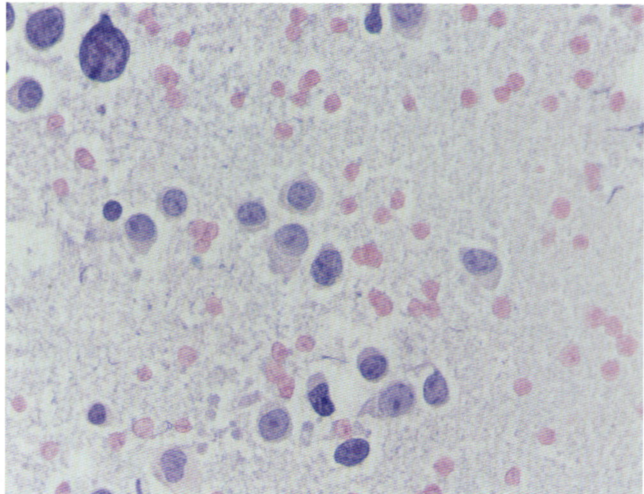

Fig. 10.16. Non-Hodgkin's lymphoma of the cervix. Pap, 60×.

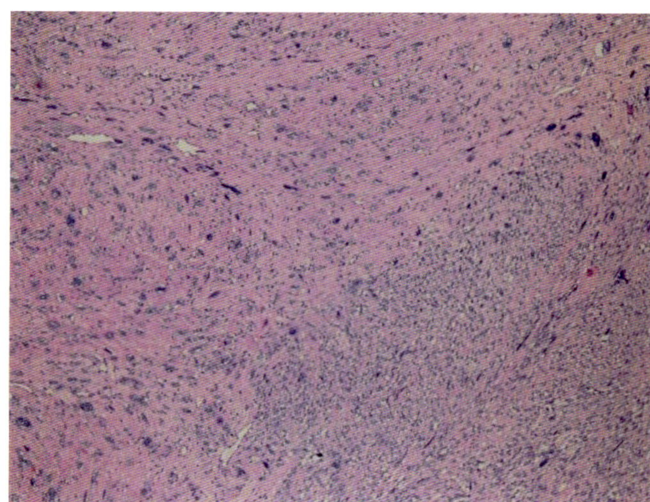

Fig. 10.18. Histopathology of leiomyosarcoma. Histology: HE, 10×.

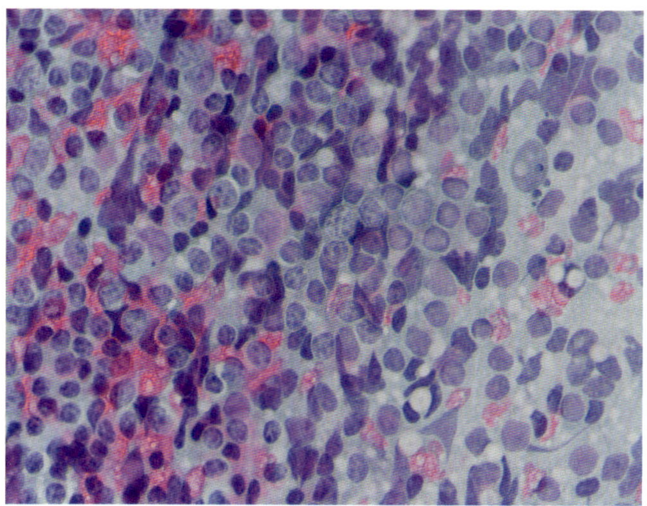

Fig. 10.17. Smear of follicular cervicitis. Pap, 60×.

invasion. The presence of stellate cells favors a cytological diagnosis of ESS [33].

Benign Lesions

Smears of *follicular cervicitis* contain benign reactive lymphocytes and plasma cells (fig. 10.17). Occasional cellular and nuclear moulding seen in ESS help in the differentiation [145].

Finally, ESS may be difficult to distinguish from stromal endometriosis of the cervix in cytological smears. In this condition, smears contain only closely packed endometrial stromal cells of benign type and no epithelial endometrial cells. A hypercellular smear of benign stromal cells is a clue [34, 98].

Leiomyosarcoma

Concept. A malignant tumor of neoplastic cells showing smooth muscle differentiation.

Clinical Features. LMS is the commonest pure uterine sarcoma and represents over 1% of all malignant uterine tumors. It occurs in the perimenopausal age group, nearly a decade later than leiomyoma [79, 204]. It is not usually associated with leiomyoma. However, rapid growth in size of the uterus of a postmenopausal woman suggests the possibility of LMS. Vaginal bleeding and an irregularly enlarged uterus are the commonest symptoms.

LMS are highly malignant tumors. The prognosis is mainly related to the extent of recurrence [79].

Histopathology. The histological pattern of LMS is of fascicles of spindle-shaped, ovoid or rounded cells, which have the morphologic, ultrastructural and immunocyto-chemical characteristics of smooth muscle cells expressing actin and desmin. The cells have abundant eosinophilic cytoplasm and fusiform hyperchromatic nuclei with coarse chromatin, macronucleoli and increased mitotic activity [79] (fig. 10.18).

Cytopathology. LMS do not usually exfoliate cells, except when ulcerated or necrotic. This fact makes cytological diagnosis on a Pap smear difficult. A diagnosis is only achieved in 15% of cases [219]. Neoplastic cells seen in smears, mainly of EBT, usually show the following features:

Cytopathology of the Non-Epithelial
Malignant Tumors of the Uterine Corpus

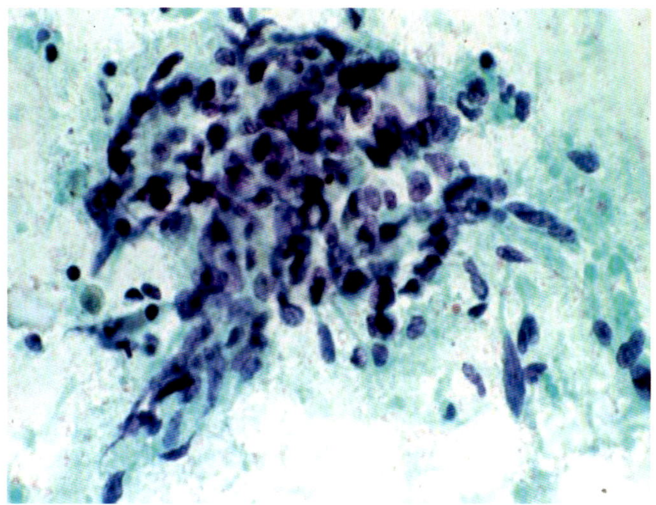

Fig. 10.19. Cytopathology of leiomyosarcoma: large spindle cells. Pap, 40×.

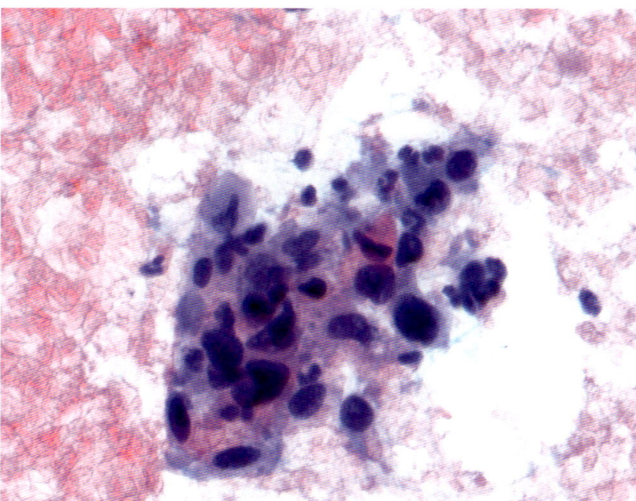

Fig. 10.21. Squamous cell carcinoma of the cervix. Pap, 60×.

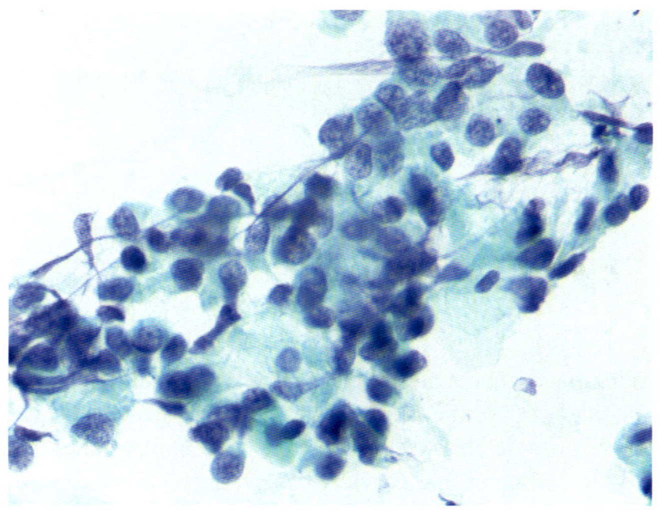

Fig. 10.20. Leiomyosarcoma: anisonucleosis. Pap, 60×.

Table 10.3. Leiomyosarcoma cytological differential diagnosis

Malignant tumors
– Squamous cell carcinoma
– Malignant müllerian mixed tumors
– Malignant melanoma

Benign lesions
– Reparative and regenerative epithelial cells. Leiomyoma

Shedding: Large pleomorphic spindle cells, mostly isolated, but whorls of tumor cells can be found [148] (fig. 10.19).

Cytoplasm: Abundant fibrillar cytoplasm, eosinophilic or amphophilic.

Nuclei: Ovoid, cigar-shaped nuclei with blunt ends, coarse chromatin and irregular nucleoli, varying in shape, size and numbers (fig. 10.20).

Multinucleated giant cells are often found.

Background: There is usually a bloody and 'dirty' background with many inflammatory cells but with less debris than in usual tumor diathesis [145].

Differential Diagnosis. The diagnosis of malignancy is usually easy in EBT smears of LMS. The tumor cell nuclei are pleomorphic with abnormal chromatin and mitotic figures, and there is evidence of necrosis in the background. It is more difficult to type the tumor as LMS and to distinguish it from other malignant tumors (table 10.3).

Malignant Tumors
Squamous Cell Carcinoma. Cells of keratinizing squamous lesions have dense eosinophilic cytoplasm, which is unusual in cells from a sarcoma (fig. 10.21). Sarcoma cells show more pleomorphism than squamous neoplastic cells.

Malignant Mesodermal Mixed Tumors (MMMT). Anaplastic cells similar to those of poorly-differentiated LMS are also present in MMMT. The identification of epithelial neoplastic cells in mixed tumors may help in some cases.

Malignant Melanoma. Pleomorphic malignant cells are found as in LMS. Identification of melanin pigment is the key diagnostic feature (fig. 10.22).

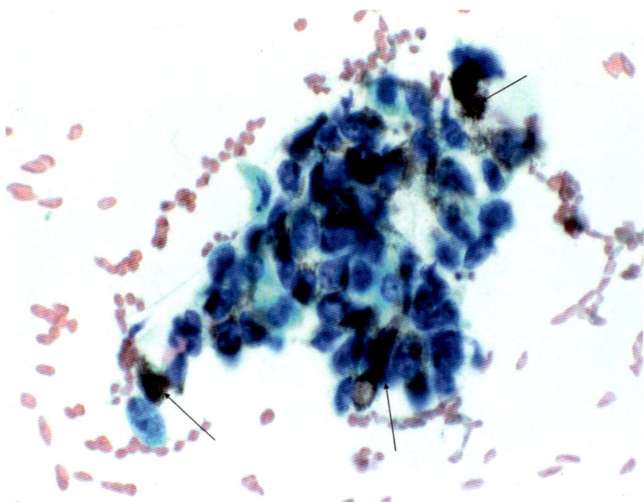

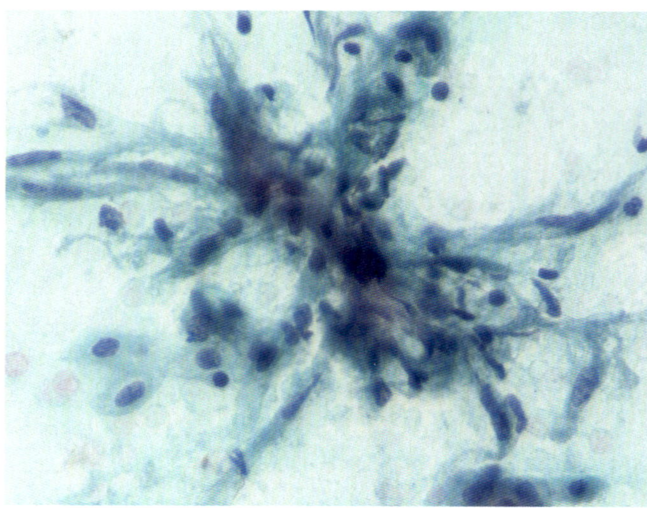

Fig. 10.22. Malignant melanoma. Melanin pigment is seen in the cytoplasm of some cells. Pap, 60×.

Fig. 10.24. Leiomyoma: worm-shaped bodies. Pap, 60×.

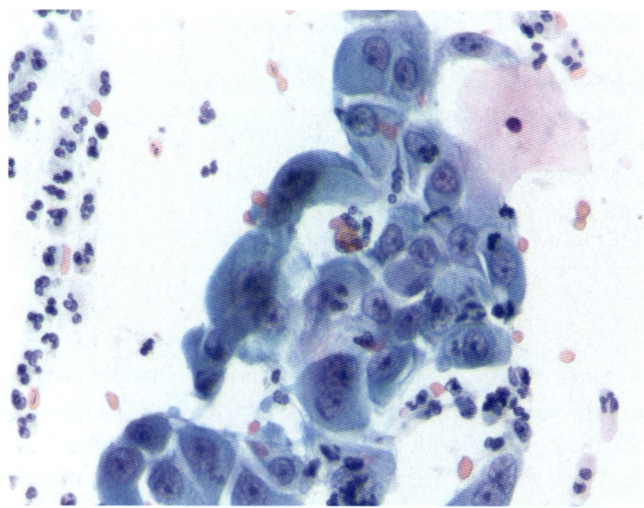

Fig. 10.23. Smear of reparative process of the cervix. Pap, 60×.

Benign Lesions
Reparative and Regenerative Cells of the Cervix. The absence of malignant nuclear features helps to prevent mistakes (fig. 10.23).

Leiomyoma. The distinction between leiomyoma (fig. 10.24) and poorly-differentiated LMS can be difficult in cytological smears in the event of necrosis and shedding, which occurs in both tumors [180]. Multinucleated cells, nuclear shape, and necrosis are key features of LMS, but it may be difficult to distinguish neoplastic cells from normal

Table 10.4. Mixed epithelial and mesenchymal tumors (WHO, 2003)

Carcinosarcoma (malignant mesodermal mixed tumors)
Adenosarcoma
Carcinofibroma
Adenofibroma
Adenomyoma:
– Atypical polyploid variant

fibrous and smooth muscle cells in some poorly-differentiated tumors [145]. Large benign necrotizing myomas may cause more considerable difficulties in particular when these lesions appear in the cervical os giving the impression of being born ('in status nascendi').

10.5. Concept of Mixed Epithelial and Mesenchymal Tumors

These are tumors of the uterine corpus which have both an epithelial and a mesenchymal component. Table 10.4 shows the 2003 WHO Classification of this group of neoplasms [127].

Carcinosarcoma
Concept. The definition of carcinosarcoma is a biphasic tumor composed of a mixture of malignant epithelial and mesenchymal components. Several synonymous terms are used: malignant mesodermal mixed tumors, MMMT and

Cytopathology of the Non-Epithelial
Malignant Tumors of the Uterine Corpus

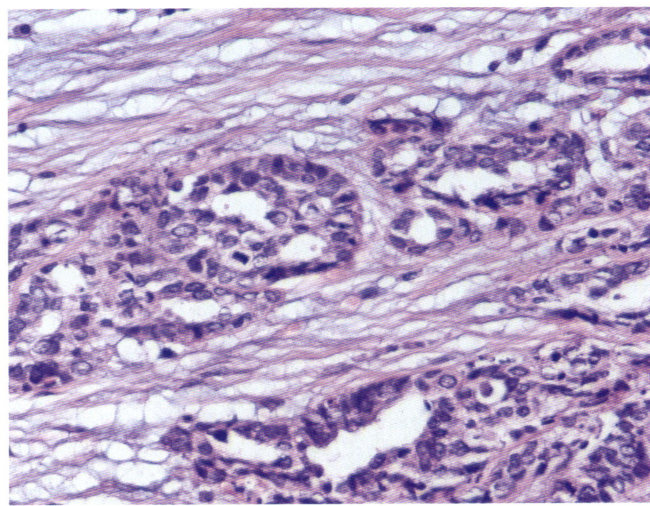

Fig. 10.25. Histopathology of carcinosarcoma, homologous type. Epithelial component is predominant in this area. HE, 40×.

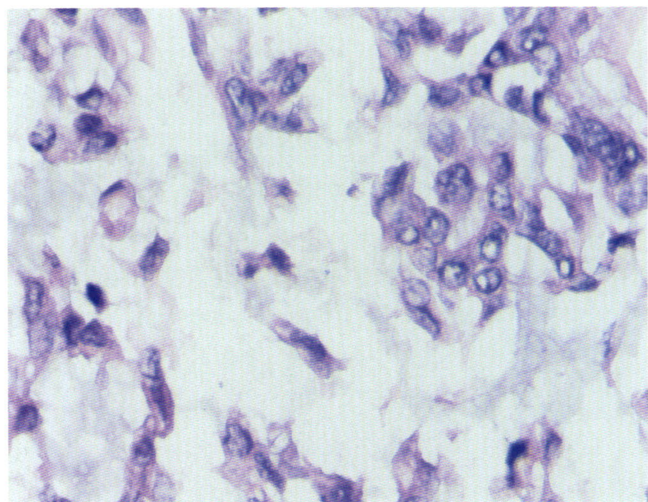

Fig. 10.26. MMMT with rhabdomyosarcomatous component. HE, 40×.

metaplastic carcinoma. These tumors are still classified as 'mixed' by convention, but there is increasing evidence that they are monoclonal and should be considered as a variant of EC (WHO, 2003), i.e. a sarcomatoid carcinoma rather than a carcinosarcoma [141, 201].

Epidemiology and Etiology. Carcinosarcoma is an uncommon, highly aggressive tumor that represents only around 5% of malignant neoplasms of the uterine corpus. It usually occurs in postmenopausal women with a median age of 65. Only less than 5% of patients are younger than 50 [150].

As mentioned in Chapter 1, an association with long-term tamoxifen therapy, mostly in patients treated for breast carcinoma, has been suggested. Up to 30% of cases have had previous pelvic radiation [151].

Clinical Features. MMMT usually presents as a polypoid growth protruding through the cervical os. Vaginal bleeding occurs which may be associated with an abdominal mass and pelvic pain. The tumors are usually aggressive and have a poor prognosis. Large series suggest that the various histological patterns of the mesenchymal elements bear no relation to the overall prognosis [79].

Diagnostic Methods

Cytology. The majority of patients with carcinosarcoma do not have abnormal cervicovaginal smears. Malignant cells appear in smears at an advanced stage of the disease when the tumor involves the lower uterine segment or the cervix with greater risk of recurrence. The sensitivity for the detection of cancer cells is low, 56–70% [27]. Better results have been obtained by EBT, but marked necrosis of a small sarcomatous component make a specific cytological diagnosis difficult, both in Pap and in EBT [158]. The difficulty is compounded by sampling error, haphazard exfoliation and cellular degeneration [27]

Imaging. Magnetic resonance imaging demonstrates an enlarged uterus with a widened endometrial cavity and deep myometrial invasion. EA needs to be ruled out. The demonstration of a large uterus with extensive myometrial invasion and ovarian or intraperitoneal spread is suggestive of carcinosarcoma.

Histological Methods. Although uterine curettage is the most important diagnostic method, a preoperative diagnosis can be difficult and over 25% of carcinosarcomas are diagnosed only after hysterectomy [79].

Histopathology

Macroscopy and Spread. Carcinosarcoma presents as a large polypoid and hemorrhagic growth involving the endometrium and myometrium. Frequently, the tumor may arise in a benign EP. Intra-abdominal and retroperitoneal metastases are commonly present.

Microscopic Examination. The MMMT contains both malignant epithelium and malignant mesenchymal elements. The malignant epithelial component can be glandular, squamous or undifferentiated. The glandular element is usually endometrioid but may also be serous or clear cell in type.

The sarcomatous component may be of a homologous type (fig. 10.25) which includes LMS, UES and EES, usually high grade. The heterologous type is composed of sarcomatous

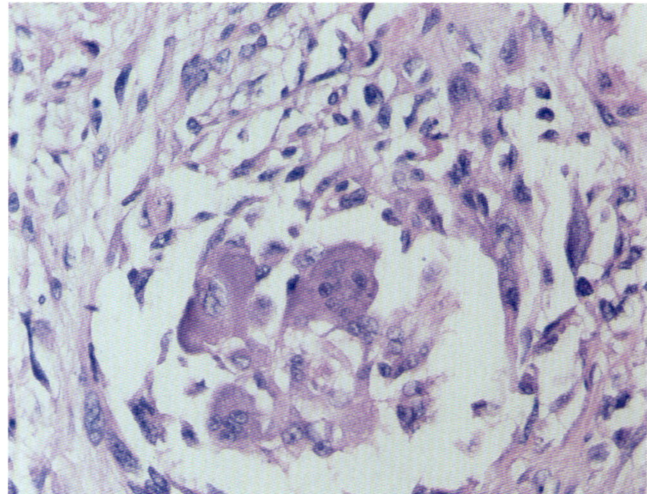

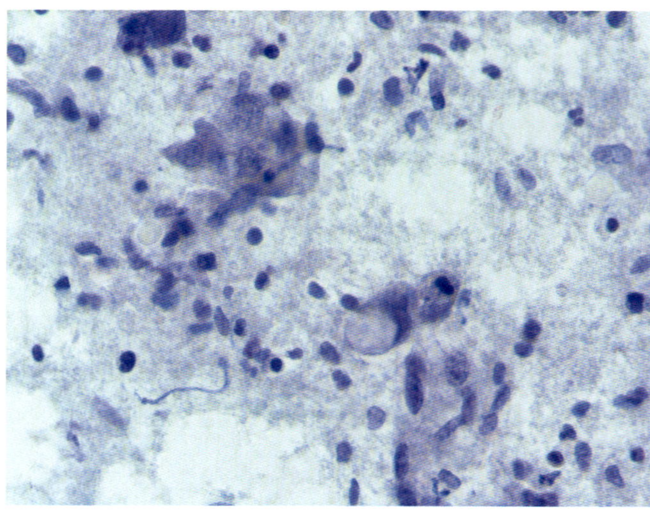

Fig. 10.27. MMT with a chondrosarcomatous component. HE, 40×.

Fig. 10.28. Cytology of heterologous carcinosarcoma with bizarre cells. Pap, 60×.

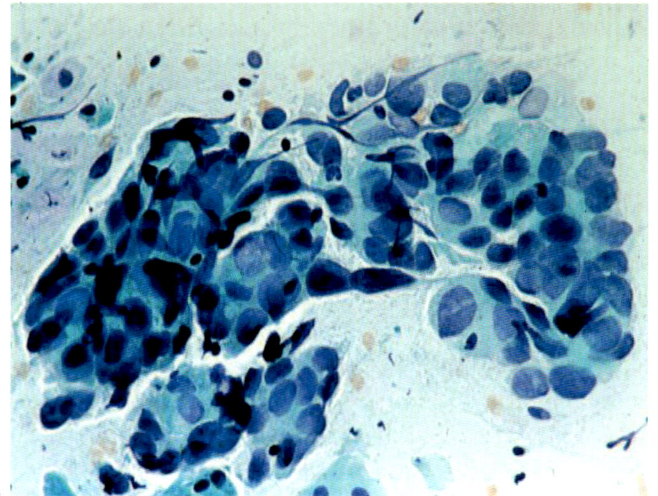

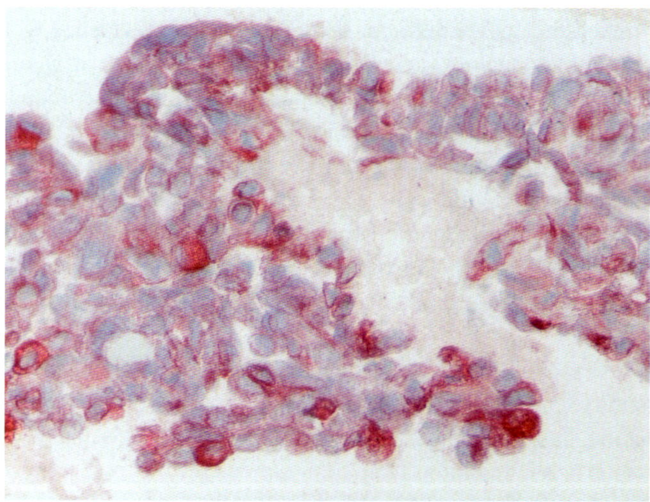

Fig. 10.29. MMMT with adenocarcinoma cells and raquetoid cells of rhabdomyosarcoma. **a** Pap, 40×. **b** Cam 5.2 ++ 60×.

tissue elements not normally seen in the uterus such as rhabdomyosarcoma (fig. 10.26), osteosarcoma, chondrosarcoma (fig. 10.27) and liposarcoma.

Immunoprofile. The epithelial component expresses cytokeratin, and the mesenchymal elements express vimentin and focally cytokeratin (fig. 10.29b). The concordance of TP53 staining of the epithelial and the mesenchymal components supports a common monoclonal origin [79].

Cytopathology

Smears of MMMT usually show a background tumor diathesis. Two types of neoplastic cells may be found. The malignant epithelial cells are usually analogous to EA, less often they may be derived from a squamous component. In the latter case, the malignant cells are similar to those of cervical squamous carcinoma, usually of large-cell non-keratinizing type. In 10–40% of cases with few sarcomatous

Cytopathology of the Non-Epithelial
Malignant Tumors of the Uterine Corpus

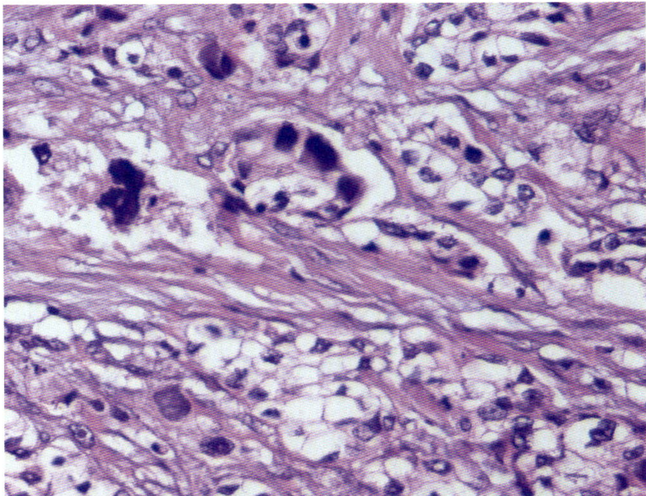

Fig. 10.30. Histopathology of the tumor of the patient in figure 10.31. HE, 40×.

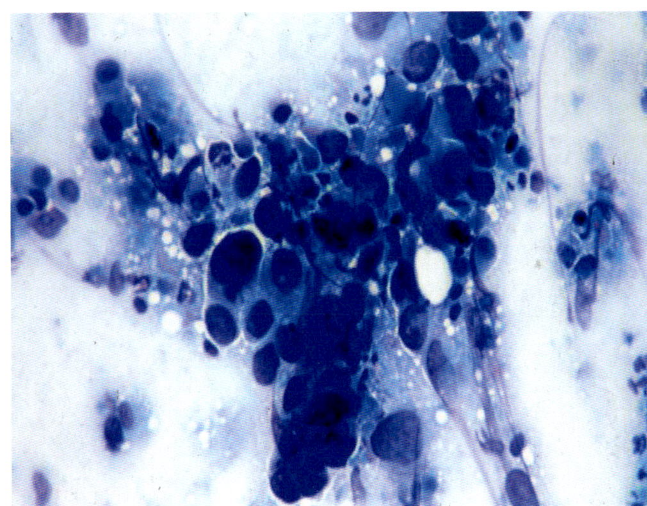

Fig. 10.32. Peritoneal wash: peritoneal metastases of MMMT. Pap, 60×.

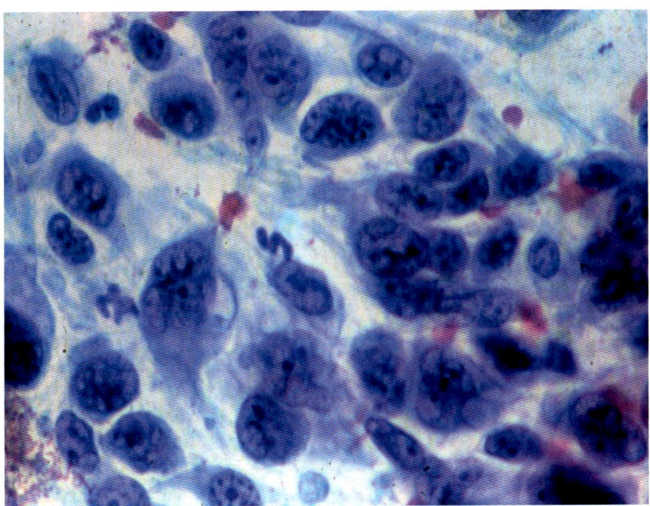

Fig. 10.31. Fine-needle aspiration cytology of a node of a patient with MMMT. Pap, 60×.

Table 10.5. Carcinosarcoma. Cytological differential diagnosis

Adenocarcinoma with squamous differentiation
Carcinoma with a desmoplastic reaction
Carcinosarcoma of other sites
Adenosarcoma
Choriocarcinoma

cells we can only report the cytomorphology as mesenchymal malignancy, but not a specific type of tumor. The mesenchymal cells are bizarre, elongated or raquetoid in shape with a lacy or fibrillar cytoplasm texture. The nuclei, sometimes multiple, are hyperchromatic and have prominent nucleoli (fig. 10.28) [51].

Some cases of MMMT exhibit some specific cytological features. If the tumor has a rhabdomyosarcomatous component, spindle and strap cells, multinucleated giant cells and cells with cross-striation may be found (fig. 10.29).

A chondrosarcomatous component may be represented by cells with semitransparent cytoplasm associated with a cartilaginous matrix. Osteoid or lipomatous components are more difficult to identify.

Cytopathology of Recurrences and Metastases

A cytological diagnosis of possible recurrent or metastatic MMMT may be considered in two different situations. There are usually no difficulties in the presence of a relevant clinical history; malignant cells of a biphasic tumor in the smear would suggest carcinosarcoma. An evaluation of specific features in a suspected tumor focus may need a fine-needle aspiration cytology procedure (fig. 10.30, 10.31). Smears show marked tumor diathesis and malignant cells which are less differentiated than those of the primary tumor (fig. 10.32). The mesenchymal component is represented by malignant giant cells and by cells showing severe degrees of anaplasia, but is only found in 50% of recurrent tumors and in 20% of metastatic tumors [141]. If there is no history available and no information about a primary tumor, it is very difficult not only to type the tumor but sometimes also to confirm malignancy in smears.

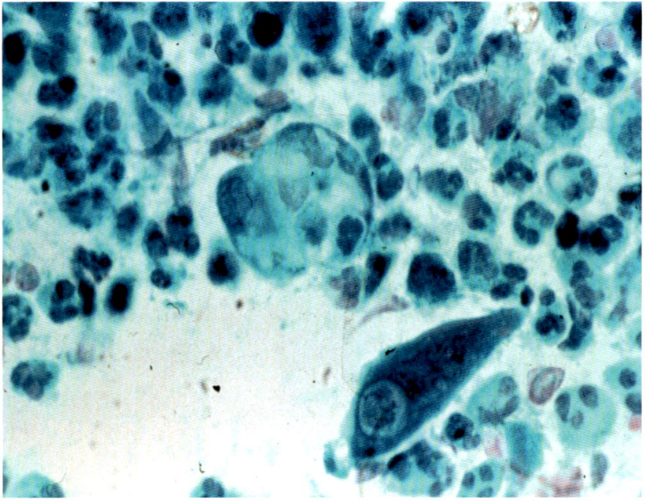

Fig. 10.33. Adenosquamous carcinoma of the cervix. Pap, 60×.

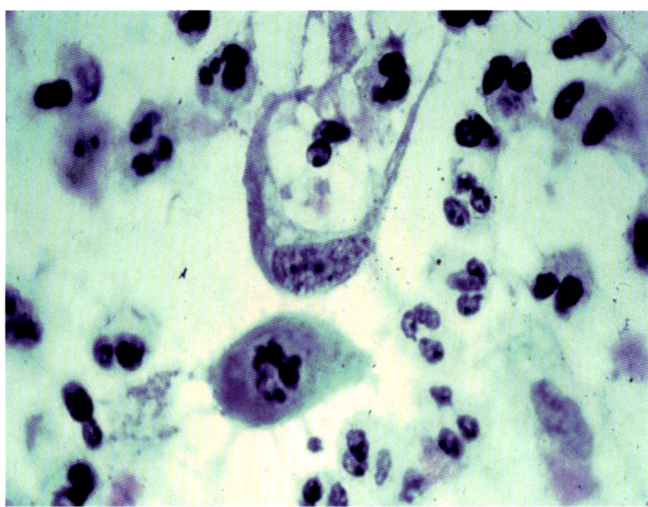

Fig. 10.35. Rhabomyosarcoma botryoides of the vulva. Pap, 60×.

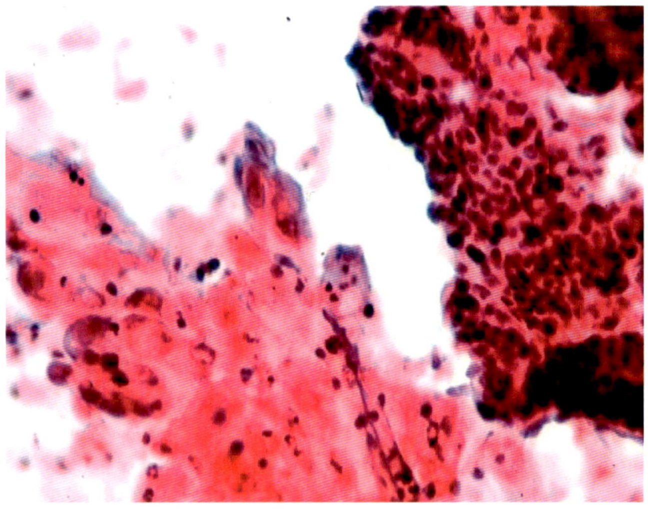

Fig. 10.34. Endometrial adenocarcinoma with squamous differentiation. Pap, 40×.

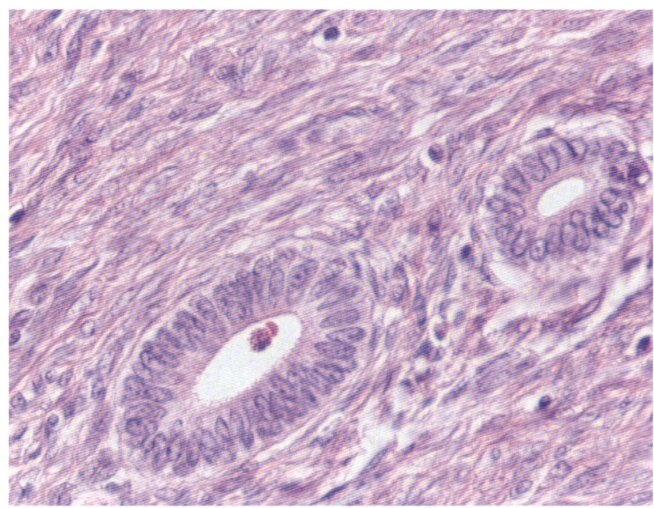

Fig. 10.36. Histopathology of adenosarcoma. HE, 40×.

Differential Diagnosis

The differential diagnosis of carcinosarcoma in cytological preparations is summarized in table 10.5.

Adenocarcinoma with Squamous Differentiation. This tumor can occur in the cervix and in the endometrium. The identification of malignant mesenchymal cells by morphology and immunocytochemistry is the key to diagnosis (figs 10.33, 10.34).

Carcinoma with a Desmoplastic Reaction. As in the previous type the smear shows only an epithelial component.

Carcinosarcoma of Other Sites. Clinical and histopathological features indicating another possible primary site are needed to suggest this possibility (fig. 10.35).

Adenosarcoma. This rare uterine tumor has a benign epithelial component, usually of an endometrial or endocervical type, associated with malignant mesenchymal elements, which may be of homologous type (ESS) or of heterologous type (rhabdomyoblast or chondroblasts) [190] (figs 10.36, 10.37).

Cytopathology of the Non-Epithelial
Malignant Tumors of the Uterine Corpus

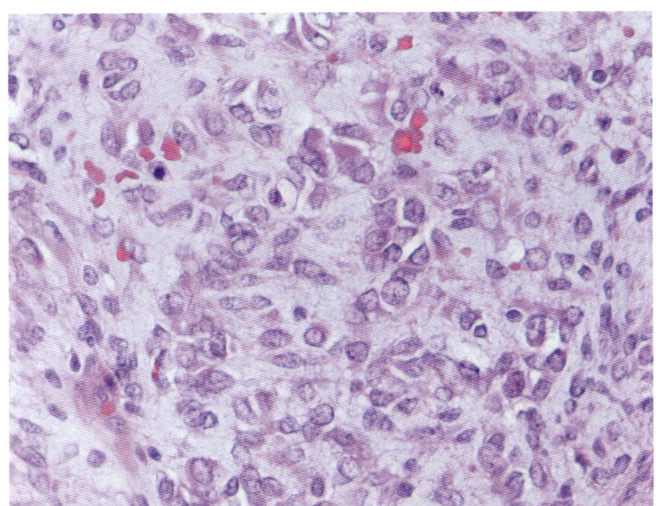

Fig. 10.37. Adenosarcoma of the uterus. HE, 40×.

Choriocarcinoma. This trophoblastic tumor does not shed cells frequently and is usually associated with a recent pregnancy. Two types of malignant cells may be identified in smears, multinucleated syncytiotrophoblastic cells and mononucleated cytotrophoblastic cells similar in size to parabasal cells but with enlarged nuclei, macronucleoli and pleomorphic shapes [148] (fig. 9.40).

References

1 Abadi MA, Barakat R, Saigo PE: Effects of tamoxifen on cervicovaginal smears from patients with breast cancer. Acta Cytol 2000; 44:141–146.
2 Alonso de Ruiz P: Endometrial cells in conventional cervical cytology. A controversy on endometrial neoplastic lesions. Satellite Symposium with SLAP XV International Congress of Cytology, Santiago de Chile, April 11–15, 2004.
3 Alvarez-Santín C, Sica A, Rodriguez MC, Feijó A, Garrido G: Microglandular hyperplasia of the uterine cervix. Cytologic diagnosis in cervical smears. Acta Cytol 1999;43:110–113.
4 Arcos de la Plaza M: La citología endometrial en España. Citología 1984;6:149–158.
5 Anastasiadis PG, Koutlaki NG, Skaphida PG, Galazios GC, Tsikouras PN, Liberis VA: Endometrial polyps: prevalence, detection, and malignant potential in women with abnormal uterine bleeding. Eur J Gynaecol Oncol 2000;21:180–183.
6 Ashfag R, Gibbons D, Vela C, Saboorian MH, Iliya F: ThinPrep Pap Test. Accuracy for glandular disease. Acta Cytol 1999;43:81–85.
7 Assikis VJ, Jordan VC: Gynecologic effects of tamoxifen and the association with endometrial carcinoma. Int J Gynecol Obstet 1995;49: 241–257.
8 Bai H, Sung CJ, Steinhoff MM: ThinPrep Pap Test promotes detection of glandular lesions of the endocervix. Diagn Cytopathol 2000;23:19–22.
9 Ben-Arie A, Goldchmit C, Laviv Y, Levy R, Caspi B, Huszar M, Dgani R, Hagay Z: The malignant potential of endometrial polyps. Eur J Obstet Gynecol Reprod Biol 2004;115: 206–210.
10 Benson JR, Pitsinis V: Update on clinical role of tamoxifen. Curr Opin Obstet Gynecol 2003;15:13–23.
11 Bean SM, Conolly K, Roberson J, Eltoum I, Chieng DC: Incidence and clinical significance of morphologically benign-appearing endometrial cells in patients age 40 years or older. Cancer Cytopathol 2006;108:39–44.
12 Bergeron C, Nogales FF, Masseroli M, Abeler V, Duvillard P, Muller-Holzner E, Pickartz H, Wells M: A multicentric European study testing the reproducibility of the WHO classification of endometrial hyperplasia with a proposal of a simplified working classification for biopsy and curettage specimens. Am J Surg Pathol 1999;23:1102–1108.
13 Bergman L, Beelen ML, Gallee MP, Hollema H, Benraadt J, Van Leeuwen FE: Risk of prognosis of endometrial cancer after tamoxifen for breast cancer. Comprehensive Cancer Centres ALERT Group. Assessment of Liver and Endometrial Cancer. Risk following Tamoxifen. Lancet 2000;356: 881–887.
14 Bettocchi S, Ceci O, Vicino M, Marello F, Impedovo L, Selvaggi L: Diagnostic inadequacy of dilatation and curettage. Fertil Steril 2001;75:803–805.
15 Bibbo M: The vakutage method in the detection of endometrial cancer and its precursors; in Wied GL, Keebler CM, Koss LG, Reagan JW (eds): Compendium on Diagnostic Cytology, ed 6. Chicago, Tutorials of Cytology, 1998, pp 213–227.
16 Bistoletti P, Hjerpe A: Routine use of endometrial cytology in clinical practice. Acta Cytol 1993;37:867–870.
17 Bjarnason K, Cerin A, Lindgren R, Weber T; Long Cycle Study Group: Adverse endometrial effects during long cycle hormone replacement therapy. Maturitas 1999;32:161–170.
18 Boman F: Pap smear and endometrial tumor. Ann Pathol 2004;24:71–72.
19 Bonfiglio TA, Clary KM: Cytology of glandular lesions in liquid-based gynecologic specimens. Workshop 4. 53rd Annual Scientific Meeting of the American Society of Cytopathology, San Diego 2005, pp 1–15.
20 Brewster WR, Monk BJ, Burger RA, Berger S, Wilczynski SP: Does human papillomavirus have a role in cancers of the uterine corpus? Gynecol Oncol 1999;75:51–54.
21 Brölmann HA, Dijkhuizen FP, Mol BW: The clinical importance of the microcurettage. Rev Gynaecol Pract 2004;4:58–64.
22 Buckley CH, Fox H: The anatomy and histology of the endometrium; in Gottlieb LS, Neville AM, Walker F (eds): Biopsy Pathology of the Endometrium. Biopsy Pathology Series 14. London, Chapman & Hall Medical, 1988, pp 11–29, 38–50,144–148.
23 Buratti E, Cefis F, Masserini M, Goisis F, Vergadoro F, Bolis G: The value of endometrial cytology in a high-risk population. Tumori 1985;71:25–28.
24 Byrne AJ: Endocyte endometrial smears in the cytodiagnosis of endometrial carcinoma. Acta Cytol 1990;34:373–378.
25 Cangiarella JF, Chhieng DC: Atypical glandular cells – an update. Diagn Cytopathol 2003;29:271–279.
26 Cardosi RJ, Florica JV: Surveillance of the endometrium in tamoxifen-treated women. Curr Opin Obstet Gynecol 2000;12:27–31.
27 Casey MB, Candill JL, Salomao DR: Cervicovaginal (Papanicolaou) smears findings in patients with malignant mixed müllerian tumors. Diagn Cytopathol 2003;28:245–249.
28 Chang A, Sandweiss L, Bose S: Cytologically benign endometrial cells in the Papanicolaou smears of postmenopausal women. Gynecol Oncol 2001;80:37–43.
29 Cherkis RC, Patten SF, Andrews TJ, Dickinson JC: Significance of normal endometrial cells detected by cervical cytology. Obstet Gynecol 1988;71:242–244.
30 Chhieng DC, Elgert P, Cohen JM, Cangiarella JF: Clinical implications of atypical glandular cells of undetermined significance, favor endometrial origin. Cancer Cytopathol 2001;93: 351–356.
31 Cibas ES: Cervical and vaginal cytology; in Ciba ES, Ducatman BS (eds): Cytology. Diagnostic Principles and Clinical Correlates, ed 2. Edinburgh, Saunders, 2003, pp 47–60.
32 Clement PB, Young RH: Endometrioid carcinoma of the uterine corpus: a review of its pathology with emphasis on recent advances and problematic aspects. Adv Anat Pathol 2002;9:145–184.
33 Clement PB, Young RH: Non-endometrioid carcinoma of the uterine corpus: a reviews of their pathology with emphasis on recent advances and problematic aspects. Adv Anat Pathol 2004;11:117–142.
34 Clement PB, Young RH, Scully RE: Stromal endometriosis of the uterine cervix. A variant of endometriosis that may simulate a sarcoma. Am J Surg Pathol 1990;14:449–455.
35 Cohen I, Rosen DJD, Shapira J, Cordoba M, Gilboa S, Altaras MM, Yigael D, Beyth Y: Endometrial changes in postmenopausal women treated with tamoxifen for breast cancer. Br J Obstet Gynecol 1993;100:567–570.
36 Cohen I: Endometrial pathologies associated with postmenopausal tamoxifen treatment. Gynecol Oncol 2004;94:256–266.
37 Connell PP, Rotmensch J, Waggoner SE, Mundt AJ: Race and clinical outcome in endometrial carcinoma. Obstet Gynecol 1999; 94:713–720.

38 Cornier E, Feintuch MJ, Delafontaine D, Thouvenin R, Bouccara L: Une nouvelle technique pour le prélèvement histologique de l'endomètre en consultation externe: la Pipelle. Gynécologie 1982;33:169.

39 Cornier E: The Pipelle: a disposable device for endometrial biopsy. Am J Obstet Gynecol 1984;148:109–110.

40 Coscia-Porrazzi LO, Maiello FM, Falco ML: The cytology of the normal cyclic endometrium. Diagn Cytopathol 1986;2:198–203.

41 Coscia-Porrazzi LO: Cytologic criteria of hyperplastic lesions in endometrial samples obtained by the Endocyte sampler. Diagn Cytopathol 1988;4:283–287.

42 Covell JL, Wilburg DC, Guidos B, Lee KR, Chhieng DC, Mody DR: Epithelial abnormalities: Glandular; in Solomon D, Nayar R (eds): The Bethesda System for Reporting Cervical Cytology, ed 2. New York, Springer, 2004, pp 123–156.

43 Cramer J, Osborne RJ: Endometrial neoplasia. Screening the high-risk patients. Am J Obstet Gynecol 1981;139:285–288.

44 Crow J, Gordon H, Hudson E: An assessment of the Mi-Mark endometrial sampling technique. J Clin Pathol 1980;33:72–80.

45 Curtin CT, Mitchell V, Curtin E: Cytology of primary squamous cell carcinoma of the endometrium. Acta Cytol 1983;27:313–316.

46 Czerwenka K, Lu Y, Heuss F, Manavi M, Kubista E: Human papillomavirus detection of endometrial carcinoma with squamous differentiation of the uterine corpus. Gynecol Oncol 1996;61:210–214.

47 Dallenbach-Hellweg G: Histopathology of the Endometrium, ed 3. Berlin, Springer, 1981, pp 22–88.

48 Davey E, Barrot A, Invig L, Chan SF, Macaskin P, Mannes P, Saville AM: Effect of study design and quality on unsatisfactory rates, cytology classification and accuracy in liquid-based versus conventional cervical cytology: a systematic review. Lancet 2006;367:122–132.

49 Del Priore G, Williams R, Harbatkin CB, Wan LS, Mittal K, Yang GCH: Endometrial brush biopsy for the diagnosis of endometrial cancer. J Reprod Med 2000;46:439–443.

50 De May RM: The cytology of pregnancy; in De May (ed): The Art and Science of Cytopathology. Chicago, ASCP Press, 1996, pp 133–137.

51 De May RM: Cytology of rare tumors, metastases, and miscellaneous findings; in De May RM (ed): The Art and Science of Cytopathology. Chicago, ASCP Press, 1996, pp 136–137.

52 Diaz-Rosario LA, Kabawat SE: Cell block preparation by inverted filter sedimentation is useful in the differential diagnosis of atypical glandular cells of undetermined significance in ThinPrep specimens. Cancer Cytopathol 2000;90:265–272.

53 Dietel M: The histological diagnosis of endometrial hyperplasia. Is there a need to simplify? Virchow Arch 2001;435:604–608.

54 Dijkhuizen FP, Mol BW, Brolmann HA, Heintz AP: The accuracy of endometrial sampling in the diagnosis of patients with endometrial carcinoma and hyperplasia: a meta-analysis. Cancer 2000;89:1765–1772.

55 Dunn JE: Geographic considerations of endometrial cancer. Gynecol Oncol 1974;2:114–121.

56 Duska LR, Garrett A, Rueda BR, Haas J, Chang Y, Fuller AF: Endometrial cancer in women 40 years old or younger. Gynecol Oncol 2001;83:388–393.

57 Elit L: Endometrial cancer. Prevention, detection, management and follow-up. Can Fam Physician 2000;46:887–892.

58 Emoto M, Tamura R, Shirota K, Hachisuga T, Kawarabayashi T: Clinical usefulness of color Doppler ultrasound in patients with endometrial hyperplasia and carcinoma. Cancer 2002;94:700–706.

59 Epstein E, Ramirez A, Skoog L Valentin L: Transvaginal sonography, saline contrast sonohysterography and hysteroscopy for the investigation of women with postmenopausal bleeding and endometrium >5 mm. Ultrasound Obstet Gynecol 2001;18:157–162.

60 Epstein E, Ramirez A, Skoog L, Valentin L: Dilatation and curettage fails to detect most focal lesions in the uterine cavity in women with postmenopausal bleeding. Acta Obstet Gynecol Scand 2001;80:1131–1136.

61 Ferency A, Gelfand MM: Outpatients endometrial sampling with Endocyte: comparative study of the effectiveness with endometrial biopsy. Obstet Gynecol 1984;63:295–302.

62 Fishman A, Friedman JA, Kaplan AL: Synchronous endometrial and ovarian cancer in young woman taking oral contraception. Eur J Gynecol Oncol 1995;16:346–348.

63 Fox H, Buckley CM: The endometrial hyperplasias and their relationship to endometrial neoplasia. Histopathology 1982;6:493–510.

64 Franco LF: Epidemiology of uterine cancers; in Meisels A, Morin C (eds): Cytopathology of the Uterus, ed 2. Chicago, ASPC, 1997, pp 301–324.

65 Fukuda K, Mori M, Uchiyama M, Iwai K, Iwasaka T, Sugimori H, Yamasaki F: Preoperative cervical cytology in endometrial carcinoma and its clinicopathologic relevance. Gynecol Oncol 1999;72:273–277.

66 Gadducci A, Cosio S, Carpi A, Nicolini A, Genazzani AR: Serum tumor markers in the management of ovarian, endometrial and cervical cancer. Biomed Pharmacother 2004;58:24–38.

67 Geisler JP, Sorosky JI, Duong H, Buekers TE, Geisler MJ, Sood AK, Anderson B, Buller RE: Papillary serous carcinoma of the uterus: increased risk of subsequent or concurrent development of breast carcinoma. Gynecol Oncol 2001;83:501–503.

68 Goodman A, Zukerberg LR, Rice LW, Fuller AF, Young RH, Scully RE: Squamous cell carcinoma of the endometrium: a report of eight cases and a review of the literature. Gynecol Oncol 1996;61:54–60.

69 Grimes DA: Diagnostic dilatation and curettage: a reappraisal. Am J Obstet Gynecol 1982;142:1–6.

70 Grönroos M, Salmi TA, Vuento MH, Jalaba EA, Tykko JE, Maatela JJ, Aromaa AR, Stegberg R, Savolailen ER, Kaurantemi TV: Mass screening for endometrial cancer directed in risk groups of patients with diabetes and patients with hypertension. Cancer 1993;71:1278–1282.

71 Guerra JM, Jiménez-Ayala M, Zomeño M, Aleman J, Saiz-Pardo F: Carcinoma primitivo de trompa diagnosticado mediante citología vaginal. Acta Ginecol 1976;29:92–101.

72 Guidos BJ, Selvaggi SM: Collection of endometrial adenocarcinoma with the ThinPrep Pap test. Diagn Cytopathol 2000;23:260–265.

73 Gupta D, Balsara G: Extrauterine malignancies; role of Pap smears in diagnosis and management. Acta Cytol 1999;43:806–813.

74 Hachisuga T, Saito T, Kigawa J, Ohwada M, Yamazawa K, Yasue A, Iwasaka T, Suglyama T, Kita T, Nagali N: Clinicopathologic study of 56 patients with endometrial cancer during or after adjuvant tamoxifen use for their breast cancers. Gynecol Oncol 2004;95:139–144.

75 Hannaford P: Health consequences of combined oral contraceptives. Br Med Bull 2000;56:749–760.

76 Heaton RB, Harris TF, Larson D, Henry MR: Glandular cells derived from direct sampling of the lower uterine segment in patients status post-cervical cone biopsy. A diagnostic dilemma. Am J Clin Pathol 1996;106:511–516.

77 Hecht JL, Ince TA, Baak J PA, Baker HE, Ogden MW, Mutter GL: Prediction of endometrial carcinoma by subjective endometrial intraepithelial neoplasia diagnosis. Mod Pathol 2004;10:1–7.

78 Hendrickson M, Martinez A, Ross J, Kempson R, Eifel P: Uterine papillary serous carcinoma. A highly malignant form of endometrial adenocarcinoma. Am J Surg Pathol 1982;6:93–108.

79 Hendrickson MR, Tavassoli FA, Kempson RL, McCluggage WG, Haller U, Kubik-Huch RA: Mesenchymal tumours and related lesions; in Tavassoli FA, Devilec P (eds): Tumours of the Breast and Female Genital Organs. WHO Classification of Tumours. Lyon, IARC Press, 2003, pp 233–244.

80 Hoffman K, Nekhlyudov L, Deligdisch L: Endometrial carcinoma in elderly women. Gynecol Oncol 1995;58:198–201.

81 Houissa-Vuong S, Catanzano-Laroudie M, Baviera E, Balaton A, Galet B, Gedeon I, Vuong PN: Primary squamous cell carcinoma of the endometrium: case history, pathologic findings and discussion. Diagn Cytopathol 2002;27:291–293.

82 Hording U, Daugaard S, Visteldt J: Adenocarcinoma of the cervix and adenocarcinoma of the endometrium: distinction with PCR-mediated detection of HPV DNA. APMIS 1997;105:313–316.

83 Horwitz RI, Feinstein AR, Horwitz SM, Robboy SJ: Necropsy diagnosis of endometrial cancer and detection-bias in case/control studies. Lancet 1981;2:66–68.

84 Im DD, Shah KV, Rosenshein NB: Report of three new cases of squamous carcinoma of the endometrium with emphasis in the HPV status. Gynecol Oncol 1995;56:464–469.

85 Irvin WP, Rice LW, Bereowitz RS: Advances in the management of endometrial adenocarcinoma. A review. J Reprod Med 2002;47:173–189.

86 Ito E, Saito T, Suzuki T, Fujii M, Kudo R: Cytology of vaginal and uterine sarcomas. Acta Cytol 2004;48:601–607.

87 Jensen JA, Jensen JG: Abrasion of the uterine mucosa by aspiration. Preliminary report (in Danish). Ugeskr Laeger 1968;130:2124–2127.

88 Jick SS, Walker AM, Jick H: Oral contraceptives and endometrial cancer. Obstet Gynecol 1993;82:931–935.

89 Jiménez-Ayala M: Cytopathology of endometrial hyperplasias. A new classification based on the European pathologists concept. Satellite Symposium with Club Arias-Stella (SLAP). XV International Congress of Cytology, Santiago de Chile 2004.

90 Jiménez-Ayala M, Vilaplana E, Becerro de Bengoa C, Zomeño M, Granados M: Technique d'aspiration endometriale par la canule de Medhosa. Rev Cytol Clin 1973;4:15–22.

91 Jiménez-Ayala M, Vilaplana E, Becerro de Bengoa C, Zomeño M, Moreno S, Granados M: Endometrial and endocervical brushing techniques with a Medhosa cannula. Acta Cytol 1975;19:557–563.

92 Jiménez-Ayala M: Endometrial cytology: yesterday, today, tomorrow. Goldblatt Lecture. XII International Congress of Cytology, Madrid 1995.

93 Jiménez-Ayala M: Endometrial cytology. Invited Lecture. XIV International Congress of Cytology, Amsterdam 2001.

94 Jiménez-Ayala M, Jiménez-Ayala B: Introduction. Value of endometrial cytology. Panel on Endometrial Adenocarcinoma. Prevention and Early Diagnosis. XV International Congress of Cytology, Santiago de Chile 2004.

95 Jiménez-Ayala M: Endometrio: lesiones malignas. Diagnóstico diferencial. Citología 1994;2:21–26.

96 Jiménez-Ayala M, Martínez Cabruja R, Esteban ML, Chinchilla C: Serous surface papillary carcinoma of the ovary metastatic to a cervical polyp. A case report. Acta Cytol 1996;40:765–769.

97 Jiménez-Ayala M: Citopatología endometrial maligna. Adenocarcinoma extrauterino. XXX Curso Internacional de Citología Clínica, Madrid 2000: Hospital General Universitario Gregorio Marañón.

98 Jiménez-Ayala M, Lacruz C, Lecona M, Rodríguez Costa J, Rodríguez C, Velasco A, Agustín D, Andrés A: Diagnósticos citológicos de la endometriosis cervical uterina. Revisión de la literatura y presentación de tres casos. Citología 1989;11:93–101.

99 Jiménez-Ayala M, Jiménez-Ayala Portillo B: Citopatología glandular del endocérvix. Diagnóstico diferencial. Rev Esp Patol 2003;36:11–20.

100 Jiménez-Ayala M: Endometrial cytology. Invited Lecture. XIV International Congress of Cytology, Amsterdam 2001.

101 Jobo T: Cytological findings of early stage of endometrial adenocarcinoma. Panel on Endometrial Adenocarcinoma. Prevention and Early Diagnosis. XV International Congress of Cytology, Santiago de Chile 2004.

102 Johnson JE, Rahemtulla A: Endocervical glandular neoplasia and its mimics in ThinPrep Pap tests. A descriptive study. Acta Cytol 1999;43:369–375.

103 Karlsson B, Granberg S, Wikland M, Ylostalo P, Torvid K, Marsal K, Valentin L: Transvaginal ultrasonography of the endometrium in women with postmenopausal bleeding – a Nordic multicenter study. Am J Obstet Gynecol 1995;172:1488–1494.

104 Kawara K, Yamada M, Jimbo H, Shirai T, Takahashi M, Sano Y, Shiromizu K: Diagnostic usefulness of aspiration cytology endometrial cancer. Cases with normal curettage findings. Acta Cytol 2005;49:507–512.

105 Koonings PP, Moyer DL, Grimes DA: A randomized clinical trial comparing Pipelle and Tis-U-Trap for endometrial biopsy. Obstet Gynecol 1990;75:293–295.

106 Koss LG, Melamed HR (eds): Koss' Diagnostic Cytology and Its Histopathological Basis, ed 5. Philadelphia, Lippincott Williams & Wilkins, 2006.

107 Koss LG, Schreiber K, Oberlander SG, Moussouris HF, Lesser M: Detection of endometrial carcinoma and hyperplasia in asymptomatic women. Obstet Gynecol 1984;64:1–11.

108 Kriseman MM: Description of a new disposable uterine sampler (the Acurrette) for endometrial cytology and histology. S Afr Med J 1982;61:107–108.

109 Kufahl J, Pedersen I, Eriksen PS, Helkjer PE, Larsen LG, Jensen KL, Nully P, Philipsen T, Wahlin A: Transvaginal ultrasound, endometrial cytology sampled by Gynoscann and histology obtained by Uterine Explora Curette compared to the histology of the uterine specimen. Acta Obstet Gynecol Scand 1997;76:790–796.

110 Kupesic S, Bekavac I, Bjelos D, Kurjak A; Assessment of endometrial receptivity by transvaginal color Doppler and three-dimensional power Doppler ultrasonography in patients undergoing in vitro fertilization procedures. J Ultrasound Med 2001;20:125–134.

111 Kurman RJ, Zaino RJ, Norris HJ: Endometrial carcinoma; in Kurtman RJ (ed): Blaustein's Pathology of the Female Genital Tract. New York, Springer, 1944, pp 279–326.

112 Kurman RJ, Solomon D: The Bethesda System for reporting cervical/vaginal cytology diagnosis. New York, Springer, 1994.

113 Kyroudi A, Papaefthimiou M, Symiakaki H, Mentzelopoulou P, Voulgaris Z, Karakitsos P: Increasing diagnostic accuracy with a cell block preparation from thin-layer endometrial cytology. Acta Cytol 2006;50:63–69.

114 Kyroudi A, Papaetthimion M, Symiakaki H, Mentzelopoulou P, Voulgaris Z, Karakitsos P: Increasing diagnostic accuracy with a cell-block preparation from thin-layer endometrial cytology. A feasibility study. Acta Cytol 2006;50:63–69.

115 Labbé S: Cytology of malignant endometrial tumors (in French). Arch Anat Cytol Pathol 1997;45:269–279.

116 La Polla JP, Nicosia S, McCurdy C, Songster C, Ruffolo E, Roberts WS, Hoffman MS, Florica JV, Canavagh D: Experience with the Endopap device for the cytologic detection of uterine cancer and its precursors: a comparison of the Endopap with fractional curettage or hysterectomy. Am J Obstet Gynecol 1990;163:1055–1059.

117 Larson DM, Johnson KK, Broste SK, Krawisz BR, Kresl JJ: Comparison of D&C and office endometrial biopsy in predicting final histopathologic grade in endometrial cancer. Obstet Gynecol 1995;86:38–42.

118 Larson DM, Krawisz BR, Johnson KK, Broste SK: Comparison of the Z-sampler and Novak endometrial biopsy instruments for in-office diagnosis of endometrial cancer. Gynaecol Oncol 1994;54:64–67.

119 Le Bouedec G, Penault-Llorca F, de Latour M, Tortochaux J, Dauplat J: Mixed müllerian tumours of the endometrium. About four cases developed on tamoxifen treatment. Gynecol Obstet Fertil 2003;9:733–738.

120 Lipscomb GH, Lopatine SM, Stovall TG, Ling FW: A randomized comparison of the Pipelle, Accurette, and Explora endometrial sampling devices. Am J Obstet Gynecol 1994;170:591–594.

121 Maksem JA: Performance characteristics of the Indiana University Medical Center Endometrial Sampler (Tao Brush) in an outpatient office setting, first year's outcomes: recognizing histological patterns in cytologic preparations of endometrial brushing. Diagn Cytopathol 2000;22:186–195.

122 Machado F, Moreno J, Carazo M, Leon J, Fiol G, Serna R: Accuracy of endometrial biopsy with the Cornier Pipelle for diagnosis of endometrial cancer and atypical hyperplasia. Eur J Gynaecol Oncol 2003;24:279–281.

123 Mathelin C, Walter P, Gharbi M, Viville B, Gairar B, Brettes JP: Is endometrial cytology of any use? Eur J Cancer 1998;34:358–359.

124 Mathelin C, Youssef C, Annane K, Brettes JP, Bellocq JP, Walter P: Endometrial brush cytology in the surveillance of postmenopausal patients under tamoxifen: a prospective longitudinal study. Eur J Obstet Gynecol Reprod Biol 2007;132:126–128.

125 Markley RL, Milan AR: Simplified endometrial testing by the Milan-Markley technic. South Med J 1979;72:452–455.

126 McCluggage WG, Abdulkader M, Price JH, Kelehan P, Hamilton S, Beattie J, Al-Nafussi A: Uterine carcinosarcomas in patients receiving tamoxifen. A report of 19 cases. Int J Gynecol Cancer 2000;10:280–284.

127 McCluggage WG, Haller U, Kurman RJ, Kubik-Huch, RA: Mixed epithelial and mesenchymal tumours; in Tavassoli FA, Devilec P (eds): Tumours of the Breast and Female Genital Organs. WHO Classification of Tumours. Lyon, IARC Press, 2003, pp 245–249.

128 Meisels A, Fortier M, Jolicoeur C: Endometrial hyperplasia and neoplasia. Cytologic screening with the Endopap endometrial sampler. J Reprod Med 1983;28:309–313.

129 Meisels A, Morin C: Endometrial cytopathology; in Johnston WW (ed): Cytopathology of the Uterus, ed 2. Chicago, ASCP, 1997, pp 277–300.

130 Meisels A, Jolicoeur C: Criteria for the cytologic assessment of hyperplasias in endometrial samples obtained by Endopap endometrial sampler. Acta Cytol 1985;29:297–303.

131 Meisels A, Morin C: Modern Uterine Cytopathology. Chicago, ASCP Press, 2007.

132 Mencaglia L, Hamou JE: Manual de histeroscopia diagnóstica y quirúrgica. Tuttlingen, Endo-Press, 2001.

133 Mencaglia L, Valle RF, Perino A, Gilardi G: Endometrial carcinoma and its precursors: early detection and treatment. Int J Gynecol Obstet 1990;31:107–116.

134 Milan AR, Markley RL: Endometrial cytology by a new technic. Obstet Gynecol 1973;42:469–475.

135 Minucci D, Torrisi B, Castagnoli N, Lovato N, Febbraro R: Cytological evaluation of endometrial hyperplasia in relation to histological pictures. Eur J Gynecol Oncol 1984;2:119–124.

136 Mishell DR, Kaunitz AM: Devices for endometrial sampling. A comparison. J Reprod Med 1998;43:180–184.

137 Mody DR: Glandular lesions in cervicovaginal cytology: conventional, ThinPrep and SurePath. Microscopic Tutorial 10. 53rd Annual Scientific Meeting of the American Society and Cytopathology, San Diego 2005, pp 1–15.

138 Moriarty AT, Cibas ES: Endometrial cells: the how and when of reporting; in Solomon D, Nayar R (eds): Bethesda System for Reporting Cervical Cytology, ed 2. New York, Springer, 2004, pp 57–65.

139 Montz FJ: Significance of 'normal' endometrial cells in cervical cytology from asymptomatic postmenopausal women receiving hormonal replacement therapy. Gynecol Oncol 2001;81:33–39.

140 Mount SL, Wegner EK, Eltabbakh GH, Olmstead JI, Drejet AE: Significant increase of benign endometrial cells on Papanicolaou smears in women using hormone replacement therapy. Obstet Gynecol 2002;100: 445–450.

141 Mourad WA, Sneige N, Katz RL, Caraway NP, Fanning TV: Fine-needle aspiration cytology of recurrent and metastatic mixed mesodermal tumors. Diagn Cytopathol 1994;11:328–332.

142 Mutter GL; The Endometrial Collaborative Group: Endometrial intraepithelial neoplasia (EIN): will it bring order to chaos? Gynecol Oncol 2000;76:287–290.

143 Mutter GL: Histopathology of genetically defined endometrial precancers. ISGP Symposium on Endometrial Hyperplasia. Int J Gynecol Pathol 2000;19:301–309.

144 Nagai N, Uebaba Y, Oshita T, Sakata K, Murakami J, Shigemasa K, Ohama K: Endometrial cytodiagnosis using a new Softcyte versus a conventional Endocyte. Oncol Rep 2002;9:483–487.

145 Naib ZM: Other genital and ovarian neoplasms; in Naib ZM (ed): Cytopathology, ed 4. Boston, Little, Brown, 1996, pp 181–198.

146 Namig AL: Chronic endometritis: an added diagnostic value to Pap smear. Diagn Cytopathol 2004;31:397.

147 Nassar A, Fleisher SR, Nasuti JF: Value of histiocyte detection in Pap smear for predicting endometrial pathology. Acta Cytol 2003;47:762–767.

148 Ng ABP, Abdul-Karim FW: Extrauterine and non-epithelial uterine tumours; in Gray W (ed): Diagnostic Cytopathology. Edinburgh, Churchill Livingstone, 1995, pp 801–809.

149 Ng ABP, Abdul-Karim FW: Normal endometrium, reactive and inflammatory conditions; in Gray W (ed): Diagnostic Cytopathology. Edinburgh, Churchill Livingstone, 1995, pp 777–781.

150 Nguyen GK, Redburn J: Endometrial cytology by direct sampling. Its value and limitations in the diagnosis of endometrial lesions; in Rosen PP, Fechner RE (eds): Pathology Annual, Part 2. Stamford, Appleton & Lange, 1995, vol 30, pp 179–202.

151 Nguyen G, Kline TS: Essentials of Cytology. An Atlas. New York, Igaku-Shoin, 1993.

152 Nishimura Y, Watanabe J, Jobo T, Hattori M, Arai T, Kuramoto H: Cytologic scoring of endometrioid adenocarcinoma of the endometrium. Cancer 2005;105:8–12.

153 Noda S: A correct procedure to detect endometrial cancer (in Japanese). Obstet Gynecol 1989;58:56–63.

154 Nogales F, Bergeron C: A controversy on endometrial neoplastic lesions. histopathological bases for the controversy. Satellite Symposium with Club Arias-Stella (SLAP). XV International Congress of Cytology, Santiago de Chile 2004.

155 Nomenclatura Citológica SEC. Informes citológicos de endometrio. Citología 1989;11:243–248.

156 Norimatsu Y, Shimizu K, Kobayashi TK, Moriya T, Tsukayama C, Miyake Y, Ohno E: Cellular features of endometrial hyperplasia and well-differentiated adenocarcinoma using the Endocyte sampler. Diagnostic criteria based on the cytoarchitecture of tissue fragments. Cancer Cytopathol 2006;108: 77–85.

157 Novak E: A suction-curet apparatus for endometrial biopsy. JAMA 1935;104:1497–1498.

158 Oda K, Okada S, Wei T, Shirai T, Takahashi M, Sano Y, Shiromizu K: Cytodiagnostic problems in uterine sarcoma. Analysis according to a novel classification of tumour growth types. Acta Cytol 2004;48:181–186.

159 Ohno M, Shiina Y, Sakuma K, Inoue H: Method of producing tissue sections from endometrial scrapings. Cytopathology 2002;13:46–53.

160 Ohno E: Endometrial cytology. Priming Biomed 2004;1:26–37.

161 O'Leary J, Landers RJ, Crowley M, Healy I, O'Donovan M, Healy V, Kealy WF, Hogan J, Doyle CT: Human papillomavirus and mixed epithelial tumors of the endometrium. Hum Pathol 1998;29:383–389.

162 Ohkawara S, Jobo T, Sato R, Kuramoto H: Comparison of endometrial carcinoma coexisting with and without endometrial hyperplasia. Eur J Gynaecol Oncol 2000;21: 573–577.

163 Opjorden SL, Caudill JL, Humphrey SK, Salomao DR: Small cells in cervical-vaginal smears of patients treated with tamoxifen. Cancer Cytopathol 2001;93:23–28.

164 Padubidri V, Baijal L, Prakash P, Chandra K: The detection of endometrial tuberculosis in cases of infertility by uterine aspiration cytology. Acta Cytol 1980;24:319–324.

165 Palermo VG: Interpretation of endometrium obtained by the Endopap sampler and a clinic study of its use. Diagn Cytopathol 1985;1: 15–12.

166 Papaefthimiou M, Symiakaki H, Mentzelopoulou P, Giahnaki AE, Voulgaris Z, Diakomanolis E, Jyroudes A, Karakitsos P: The role of liquid-based cytology associated with curettage in the investigation of endometrial lesions from postmenopausal women. Diagn Cytopathol 2005;16: 32–39.

167 Papanicolaou GN: Atlas of Exfoliative Cytology. Cambridge/MA, Commonwealth Fund by Harvard University Press, 1963, pp 3–12.

168 Pettersson B, Adami HO, Lindgren A, Hesselius I: Endometrial polyps and hyperplasia as risk factors for endometrial carcinoma. A case-control study of curettage specimens. Acta Obstet Gynecol Scand 1985;64:653–659.

169 Porrazzi LC, Quarto F, Maiello FM, De Falco ML, Antonucci T: The value of endometrial cytology by scraping in 1,798 cases. Screening in asymptomatic women and diagnosis in symptomatic ones. Diagn Cytopathol 1987;3:112–120.

170 Prat J: Histological diagnosis in endometrial hyperplasia. Virchow Arch 2002;441: 306–307.

171 Proca D, Keyhani-Rofagha S, Copeland LJ, Hameed A: Exfoliative cytology of neuroendocrine small cell carcinoma of the endometrium. Acta Cytol 1998;42: 978–982.

172 Raab SS: Can glandular lesions be diagnosed in Pap smear cytology? Diagn Cytopathol 2000;23:127–133.

173 Reagan JW, Ng ABP: Normal cells of endometrial origin; in Reagan JW, Ng ABP (eds): The Cells of Uterine Adenocarcinoma. Monogr Clin Cytol. Basel, Karger, 1965, vol 1, pp 11–19.

174 Ronnett BM, Manos MM, Ransley IE, Fetterman BJ, Kinney WF, Hurley LB: Atypical glandular cells of undetermined significance (AGUS): cytopathologic features, histopathologic results and human papillomavirus DNA detection. Hum Pathol 1999;30:816–825.

175 Rosenblatt KA, Thomas DB; WHO Collaborative Study of Neoplasia and Steroid Contraceptives: Intrauterine devices and endometrial cancer. Contraception 1996;54: 329–332.

176 Saad RS, Takei H, Lin YL, Silverman JF, Liscomb JT, Ruiz B: Clinical significance of a cytologic diagnosis of atypical glandular cells, favor endometrial origin in Pap smears. Acta Cytol 2006;50:48–54.

177 Salomâo DR, Hughes JH, Raab SS: Atypical glandular cells of undetermined significance favor endometrial origin. Criteria for separating low-grade endometrial adenocarcinoma from benign endometrial lesions. Acta Cytol 2002;46:458–464.

178 Sasagawa M, Nishino K, Honma S, Kodama S, Takahashi T: Origin of adenocarcinoma cells observed on cervical cytology. Acta Cytol 2003;97:410–414.

179 Schneider J, Centeno MM, Ausin J: Use of the Corner Pipelle as the only means of presurgical histologic diagnosis in endometrial carcinoma: agreement between initial and final histology. Eur J Gynaecol Oncol 2000;21:74–75.

180 Schneider, V: Rare lesions of the uterus; in Mesisels A, Morin C (eds): Modern Uterine Cytopathology. Chicago, ASCP Press, 2007, pp 124–135.

181 Schorge JO, Saboorian MH, Hynan L, Ashfag R: ThinPrep detection of cervical and endometrial adenocarcinoma. Cancer Cytopathol 2002;96:338–343.

182 Segadal E: Endoscann, a new endometrial cell sampler. Br J Obstet Gynaecol 1983;90:266–271.

183 SEGO: Documentos de la SEGO. Carcinoma de endometrio. Cádiz, SEGO, 1999, pp 89–138.

184 Semczuk A, Stenzel A, Baranowski W, Rozynska K, Cybulski M, Kostuch M, Jakowicki J, Wojcierowski J: Detection of human papilomavirus types 16 and 18 in human neoplastic endometrium: lack of correlation with established prognostic factors. Oncol Rep 2000;7:905–910.

185 Senkus-Konefka E, Konefka T, Jassen J: The effects of tamoxifen on the female genital tract. Cancer Treat Rev 2004;30:291–301.

186 Sherman AI, Brown S: The precursors of endometrial carcinoma. Am J Obstet Gynecol 1979;135:947–956.

187 Sherman ME, Mazur MT, Kurman RJ: Benign diseases of the endometrium; in Kurman RJ (ed): Blaustein's Pathology of the Female Genital Tract, ed 3. New York, Springer, 2002, pp 421–466.

188 Sherman ME, Devesa SS: Analysis of racial differences in incidence, survival and mortality for malignant tumours of the uterine corpus. Cancer 2003;98:176–186.

189 Shiota A, Igarashi T, Kurose T, Ohno M, Hando T: Reciprocal effects of tamoxifen on hormonal cytopathology in postmenopausal women. Acta Cytol 2002;46:499–506.

190 Shu Y-J, Ikle FA: Cytopathology of the endometrium; in Husain OAN (ed): Correlation with Histopathology. New York, McGraw-Hill, 1992.

191 Sivridis E, Giatromanolaki A: Prognostic aspects on endometrial hyperplasia and neoplasia. Virchows Arch 2001;439:118–126.

192 Silverberg SG: Problems in the differential diagnosis of endometrial hyperplasia and carcinoma. Mod Pathol 2000;13:309–327.

193 Silverberg SG, Kurtman RJ, Nogales F, Mutter GL, Kubik-Huch RA, Tavassoli FA: Epithelial tumours and related lesions; in Tavassoli FA, Devilee P (eds): Tumours of the Breast and Female Genital Organs. WHO Classification of Tumours. Lyon, IARC Press, 2003.

194 Skaarland E: New concept in diagnostic endometrial cytology: diagnostic criteria based on composition and architecture of large tissue fragments in smears. J Clin Pathol 1986;39:36–43.

195 Smith-Bindman R, Kerlikowske K, Feldstein VA, Subak L, Scheidler J, Segal M, Brand R, Grady D: Endovaginal ultrasound to exclude endometrial cancer and other endometrial abnormalities. JAMA 1998;280:1510–1517.

196 Smith RA, Bretkopt DM, Wong JY, Logrono R: Comparison of endometrial cytology to endometrial histology. Obstet Gynecol 2000;95:528.

197 Solomon D, Nayar R (eds): The Bethesda System for Reporting Cervical Cytology, ed 2. New York, Springer, 2004.

198 Sonnendecker EW, Simon GB, Sevitz H, Hofmeyr GJ: Diagnostic accuracy of the Accurette endometrial sampler. S Afr Med J 1982;61:109–113.

199 Spicer JM, Siebert I, Kruger TF: Postmenopausal bleeding: a diagnostic approach for both private and public sectors. Gynecol Obstet Invest 2006;61:174–178.

200 Stovall TG, Solomon SK, Ling FW: Endometrial sampling prior to hysterectomy. Obstet Gynecol 1989;73:405–409.

201 Tabbara SO, Cowell JL: Otras neoplasias malignas; in Solomon D, Nayar R (eds): El Sistema Bethesda para informar la citología cervical. Definiciones, criterios y notas aclaratorias. Buenos Aires, Ediciones Journal, 2005, pp 163–174.

202 Tajima M, Inamura M, Nakamura M, Sudo Y, Yamagishi K: The accuracy of endometrial cytology in the diagnosis of endometrial adenocarcinoma. Cytopathology 1998;9: 369–380.

203 Taniguchi I, Hasumi K, Kamiya M, Takahashi M, Kobayashi T, Murakami T, Endo H, Tanemura K: Endometrial cytology by Endocyte and by Masubuchi's aspiration technic – a comparable study (in Japanese). Nippon Sanka Fujinka Gakkai Zasshi 1982;34:1746–1754.

204 Tao LC: Direct intrauterine sampling: the IUMC endometrial sampler. Diagn Cytopathol 1997;17:153–159.

205 Tao LC: Cytomorphologic appearances of normal endometrial cells during different phases of the menstrual cycle: a cytologic approach to endometrial dating. Diagn Cytopathol 1995;13:95–102.

206 Tao LC: Direct intrauterine sampling in cytology; in Johnston WW (ed): Cytopathology of the Endometrium. Chicago, ASCP, 1993, pp 1–10.

207 Titus-Ernstoff L, Hatch EE, Hoover RN, Palmer J, Greenberg ER, Ricker W, Kaufman R, Noller K, Herbst AL, Colton T, Hartge P: Long-term cancer risk in women given diethylstilbestrol during pregnancy. Br J Cancer 2001;84:126–133.

208 Todo Y, Shinichirou M, Okamoto K, Takeda M, Ebina Y, Watari M, Tarashima M, Kaneuchi M, Yamamoto R, Sakuragi N: Cytological features of cervical smears in serous adenocarcinoma of the endometrium. Jpn J Clin Oncol 2003;33:636–641.

209 Tohya T, Miyazaki K, Katabuchi H, Fujisaki S, Maeyama M: Small cell carcinoma of the endometrium associated with adenosquamous carcinoma: a light and electron microscopic study. Gynecol Oncol 1986;25: 363–371.

210 Ueda M, Ueki M, Kumagai K, Ueki K, Ikeda A, Morikawa M: Clinical evaluation of the Endosearch sampler in endometrial cytology – a preliminary report. J Med 1994;25: 305–318.

211 Uvebrant M, Bergstrom H, Hansson G, Mattsson LA: Endometrial sampling using the Mi-Mark procedure as a primary routine: first year's experience. Maturitas 1989;11: 5–12.

212 Valle RF: Hysteroscopic evaluation of patients with abnormal uterine bleeding. Surg Gynecol Obstet 1981;153:521–526.

213 Van den Bosch T, Vandendael A, Wranz PAB, Lombard CJ: Endopap versus Pipelle sampling in the diagnosis of postmenopausal endometrial disease. Eur J Obstet Gynecol 1996;64:91–94.

214 Van Hoeven KH, Zaman SS, Deger RB, Artymyshyn RL: Efficacy of the Endopap sampler in detecting endometrial lesions. Acta Cytol 1996;40:900–906.

215 Vassilakos P, Wyss R, Riotton G: Cancer de l'endomètre: une nouvelle technique de dépistage cytohistologique: l'aspiration à la canule. Mèd Hyg 1974;32:1353–1355.

216 Veneti SZ, Kyrkou KA, Kittas CN, Perides AT: Efficacy of the Isaac's endometrial cell sampler in the cytologic detection of endometrial abnormalities. Acta Cytol 1984; 28:546–554.

217 Vuopala S, Klemi OJ, Maenpaa J, Salmi T: Endobrush sampling for endometrial cancer. Acta Obstet Gynecol Scand 1989;68: 345–350.

218 Walts A, Thomas P: Endometrial cells and the AutoPap system for primary screening of cervicovaginal Pap smears. Diagn Cytopathol 2002;27:232–237.

219 Wang X, Khoo U-S, Sue W, Cheung AN: Cervical and peritoneal fluid, cytology of uterine sarcoma. Acta Cytol 2002;46: 465–469.

220 Weiderpass E, Pukkala E, Vasama-Neuvonen K, Kauppinen T, Vainio H, Paakkulainen H, Boffetta P, Partanen T: Occupational exposures and cancers of the endometrium and cervix uteri in Finland. Am J Ind Med 2001;39:572–580.

221 Wen P, Abramovich C, Wang N, Knop N, Mansbacher S, Abdul-Karim FW: Significance of histiocytes on otherwise normal cervical smears from postmenopausal women. A retrospective study of 108 cases. Acta Cytol 2003;47:135–140.

222 Whittaker J, Knight B: Endometrial hyperplasia: an update and cytopathological features. Panel on Endometrial Adenocarcinoma: Prevention and Early Diagnosis. XV International Congress of Cytology, Santiago de Chile 2004.

223 Wingo PA, Tong T, Bolden S: Cancer statistics, 1995. CA Cancer J Clin 1995;45:8–30.

224 Wolinska WH, Melamed MR, de las Heras P, Delgado E: Clear cell endometrial adenocarcinoma in a young woman: report of one case detected by cytology. Gynecol Oncol 1979;8:119–129.

225 Wright CA, Leiman G, Burgess S: The cytomorphology of papillary serous carcinoma of the endometrium in cervical smears. Cancer Cytopathol 1999;87:12–18.

226 Wright TC Jr, Cox JT, Massad LS: 2001 consensus guidelines for the management of women with cervical cytological abnormalities. JAMA 2002;287:2120–2129.

References

227 Wu HH, Bryan DC, Elsheikh TM: Endometrial brush biopsy. An accurate outpatient method of detecting endometrial malignancy. J Reprod Med 2003;48:41–45.

228 Yaziji H, Gown AM: Immunohistochemical analysis of gynaecologic tumors. Int J Gynecol Pathol 2001;20:64–78.

229 Wu HH, Casto BD, Elsheikh TM: Endometrial brush biopsy. An accurate outpatient method of detecting endometrial malignancy. J Reprod Med 2003;48:41–45.

230 Zaino RJ: Endometrial hyperplasia: it is time for a quantum leap to a new classification? ISGP Symposium on Endometrial Hyperplasia. Int Gynecol Pathol 2000;19:314–321.

231 Zaino RJ, Kurman RJ, Diana Kl, Morrow CP: The utility of the revised International Federation of Gynecology and Obstetrics histologic grading of endometrial adenocarcinoma using a defined nuclear grading system. A Gynecology Oncology Group study. Cancer 1995;75:81–86.

232 Zaino RJ, Kurman RJ, Bruneto VL, Morrow CP, Bentley RC, Capellary JO, Bitterman P: Villoglandular adenocarcinoma of the uterus: a clinicopathologic study of 61 cases. A Gynecologic Oncologic Group Study. Am J Surg Pathol 1998;22:1379–1385.

233 Zarcone R, D'Apuzzo N, Sansone A, Vullo G, Monarca M: Early diagnosis of adenocarcinoma by endometrial cytology samples. Minerva Ginecol 1997;49:421–423.

Index